A Primer for Health Care Ethics
Essays for a Pluralistic Society

Second Edition

A Primer for
Health Care Ethics

Essays for a Pluralistic Society

Second Edition

Kevin O'Rourke, O.P., J.C.D., S.T.M.

GEORGETOWN UNIVERSITY PRESS/WASHINGTON, D.C.

Georgetown University Press, Washington, D.C.
© 2000 by Georgetown University Press. All rights reserved.
Printed in the United States of America

10 9 8 7 6 5 4   2009

This volume is printed on acid-free offset book paper,

Library of Congress Cataloging-in-Publication Data

A primer for health care ethics : essays for a pluralistic society / edited by Kevin
O'Rourke.—2nd ed.
     p.   cm.
  Includes index.
  ISBN 0-87840-802-9 (pbk. : alk. paper)
     1. Medical ethics. 2. Medical ethics—Case studies. I. O'Rourke, Kevin D.

R724.D3826 2000
174'.2—dc21
                                                      00-025273

Dedicated to

Charlotte Ruzicka and Donna Troy,
true friends and inspiring colleagues

Contents

Part Three
Use and Removal of Life Support   93

Part Four
Genetics   143

Part Five
Organ Donation   161

Part Nine
Artificial Generation   261

Part Ten
Special Questions   271

Introduction

This *Primer for Health Care Ethics: Essays for a Pluralistic Society* is a collection of essays originally written for students and professors at the Saint Louis University Health Sciences Center (SLUHSC) as one element of an educational program. The essays are written monthly by the staff of the Center for Health Care Ethics, often in response to questions of health care ethics being discussed in the media. At the suggestion of several of our students and colleagues, we are making the essays available to an even larger audience. The first edition of this series appeared in 1994. In this second volume, we have included some of the original essays on fundamental issues, such as the nature of health care ethics, and several that were written since the last volume was published.

The wisdom of providing ethical studies for a wide audience of readers arises from changes in our society. During the past few years, health care ethics has become "everybody's business." The ethical implications of issues such as genetic engineering, assisted suicide, advance directives for care at the time of dying, reproductive technologies, organ transplants, and the AIDS epidemic go beyond the research laboratory, the hospital, and the long-term care cater. The ethical decisions made with regard to these contemporary research and medical procedures will determine for years to come what kind of people we shall be and what type of society we shall create.

The time is far past when scientists and health care professionals were the only people responsible for ethical decisions regarding research and health care. To paraphrase the famous proverb concerning the responsibility for decisions about war, health care ethics is too important to be left in the hands of scientists and health care professionals. Thus, although we stress the responsibilities of scientists and health care professionals in these essays and articles, we realize that these issues dramatically affect all persons in society. We address these reflections to a wide spectrum of society, realizing that people with many different talents must be involved in the decision-making process that will direct medical research and health care.

Although SLUHSC is sponsored by the Society of Jesus (the Jesuits) and thus is a Catholic institution, it attracts faculty members and students from many different ethnic and religious backgrounds. The people of SLUHSC form a pluralistic community that is similar to our society at large. Hence these essays, though not in conflict with Catholic teaching, are written for a pluralistic community. Catholic teaching has traditionally depended upon sacred scripture and natural law reasoning. These essays are based on principles founded on human reason as well as faith.

Although these essays are designed for a pluralistic audience, they are not without logical foundation, principle, or moral certitude. Health care ethics founded on personal opinion, emotional reactions, or an erroneous understanding of the human person does more harm than good. These essays are based on two objective realities: the functions or needs that human persons have in common and the goals of health care as evidenced in the professional-patient relationship. Hence, these essays contain frequent references to the physiological, psychological, social, and spiritual needs and functions of human persons. Moreover, although health care in the strict sense is concerned with only the first two functions, it must respect the other two. The mutual responsibility of persons in the professional patient relationship and the desire to heal physiological and psychological functions while respecting social and spiritual values also is a theme of this volume. We draw on a very definite concept of the human person and some precise values and goals of the healing relationship that we believe have brought out the best in people in the health care professions over the centuries.

During the past few years, the types of ethical issues that health care professionals face have changed. Whereas ethical questions in the past were directed toward medical procedures (for example, informed consent, transplantation of organs, and allowing patients to die), today and in the immediate future the more prominent ethical issues in health care will be social issues: why and how to provide health care for the poor, how to preserve quality of care in the face of government controls and fiscal constraints, how to preserve the values of medicine in the face of efforts to commercialize health care, and how to choose which health care services should be covered from the many valuable services that are available. Many of these contemporary topics are treated in this collection.

Although this collection is not presented as a textbook or a model for logical progression in the science of health care ethics, we hope that it will stimulate critical thinking, promote discussion, foster a reasoned understanding of objective principles, and, above all, help people actively involved in health care—as well as people outside the profession—to ask the right questions when they face ethical issues. Efforts are underway to make this *Primer* a text for formal continuing education programs.

The essays in this volume are gathered in ten thematic sections, with no reference to the time at which they were written. Part One contains essays that examine principles and basic concepts of medical ethics for a pluralistic society. The other sections address some of the specific issues arising in various aspects of health care. References are kept to a minimum so that the gist of logical reasoning, not the weight of authority, will be the foundation of ethical argumentation. Many of the essays consider stories or issues that have been prominent in the news media. Often, we do not seek to solve the case studies because the media usually does not present all the pertinent details that are necessary to solve particular ethical issues. We do seek, however, to present principles needed to solve similar cases that arise in clinical practice or in business settings.

The authors of these essays are all past or present faculty members of the Center for Health Care Ethics at SLUHSC: Dennis Broduer, Ph.D.; Jean deBlois, C.S.J., Ph.D.; James DuBois, Ph.D.; Louise Lears, S.C., M.A.; Gerard Magill, Ph.D.; Patrick Norris, O.P., M.A.; Griffin Trotter, M.D., Ph.D., and Kevin O'Rourke, O.P, J.C.D.

We dedicate this volume to Charlotte Ruzicka—the editor of *Health Care Ethics, USA,* the quarterly journal in which these essays first appeared—and to Donna Troy, who supported our efforts and helped produce this volume.

Kevin D. O'Rourke, O.P.

Part One

Principles and Core Values

Chapter 1 _____

What Is Health Care Ethics?

Ethics is the discipline or science by which we determine which human actions are good and which are bad. If we agree that some actions are good and some are bad, it implies that there is a norm or measure for judging human actions. That is, there must be standards to which good actions will conform and to which bad actions do not conform. In this essay, we shall discuss the standards or norms by which free human actions are judged to be good or bad.

Human beings act to fulfill their needs. What are our human needs? We can enumerate many human needs—some very significant (such as food and water) and some not so significant but which make life more pleasant (such as ice cream and television). There are four needs that are most basic or fundamental:

a. physiological needs, satisfied through food and drink
b. psychological needs, satisfied through sense pleasure, rest, and relaxation
c. social needs, satisfied through family, friends, and community
d. creative or spiritual needs, satisfied through knowledge, truth, and love

To fulfill these four needs, we have powers or functions: biological, emotional, social, and creative. All the needs and their corresponding human functions are important, but creative needs and functions are most important because they direct the attainment of all human needs. Even creative functions will depend to some degree on physiological function. In sum, the functions by which we fulfill human needs are interdependent. The human functions that enable us to fulfill our needs are conceived most aptly as dimensions of a cube rather than floors of a building.

Our needs—or "drives," as they are sometimes called—motivate us to pursue objects and activities that will satisfy our fundamental needs. We call the objects or activities that fulfill our needs "goods." We know from experience that when seeking goods that will fulfill fundamental human needs, a person must be careful to fulfill those needs in a balanced manner. That is, when fulfilling a need, one must make sure that fulfilling other needs is still possible. For example, eating appetizing food fulfills my physiological and psychological needs, but if I eat too much, I may get sick and be unable to study for the chemistry examination I have tomorrow. By fulfilling my need for food in an unbalanced manner, I have made it impossible to fulfill my creative need, which is fulfilled by passing the chemistry exam. You have heard of the person who studies so intently that she injures her health. This is another example of fulfilling needs in an unbalanced manner. This need to fulfill human needs in a balanced manner is expressed in the distinction between people who live to eat and people who eat to live.

When a human act achieves the goal of fulfilling a human need in a balanced manner, we call such an action a good action. Moreover, the action is described as having value. If a human act does not fulfill a human need or fulfills a human need in an unbalanced manner, we call such actions bad actions. Thus, if a person steals food from another, he is performing a bad action because, although he may be fulfilling his physiological need, he is not fulfilling his social needs. If a person fulfills his physiological and psychological needs by drinking beer but drinks so much that he impairs his ability to drive a car safely, he is unable to fulfill his social and creative needs and hence is performing a bad action, regardless of whether other persons are injured as a result of his drunkenness.

The free judgments by which one chooses to fulfill his or her basic needs are known as ethical decisions, or decisions of conscience. When we make decisions of conscience, difficulties arise most often in regard to social needs. Our desire to fulfill our physiological, psychological, and creative needs usually involves our own well-being. To fulfill our social needs, however, we must be concerned about the well-being of others; that is, we must respect their needs and rights. Experience teaches us how difficult it is to keep the needs and rights of others in mind as we seek to fulfill our own needs. That is why society devotes so much attention to establishing justice through laws, courts, and police. We also know, however, that respecting the rights and needs of others is vitally important because it is the basis for friendship and community, peace and progress.

As we affirm that the purpose of human acts is to fulfill human needs in a balanced manner, we also affirm that when a person fails to act in a balanced manner, he is still trying to do something that he considers to be good. In other words, if a person chooses to do something that does not fulfill his needs in a balanced manner, he chooses an action that is subjectively good but objectively bad. The distinction between subjective and objective morality is most important in ethics. This distinction helps us understand the nature of good and evil. A human action that is objectively and subjectively good fulfills a person's needs in a balanced manner. An action may be objectively evil but only subjectively good. This happens when the act is only a partial or apparent good. The error in judgment that leads a person to choose an apparent good rather than a true or balanced good may be caused by an intellectual error or moral weakness. Hence, a person may choose to take the property of another, erroneously thinking it is his own property. If one is not responsible for the ignorance that disposes one to act in this way, it might be considered an evil action objectively speaking, but it is clear that the person taking the property of the other is not doing something evil insofar as the subjective order of morality is concerned. Moral weakness might cause one to choose a partial or apparent good when the opportunity to steal money without being caught causes one to neglect fulfillment of his social needs. If a person decides to steal a large sum of money, he concentrates on the good that will come to him when he has more money and thinks little about the harm that will come to the people from whom he steals the money. If the thief thinks of his victims at all, he might excuse his violation of human rights by saying, "Anyhow, they won't miss it!"

Conflicts regarding moral judgments arise when people, either because of ignorance or moral weakness, do not consider all their human needs when they make ethical decisions. When making ethical decisions in regard to health care, for example, the medical team is interested in prolonging life—a physiological good. Patients, however, may have spiritual norms they wish to fulfill. Thus, a patient who is a Jehovah's Witness will seek to fulfill her religious belief prohibiting blood transfusions even though she may die as a result of her choice. Insofar as she is concerned, she is making a good ethical decision because fulfilling her spiritual need is more important than fulfilling her physiological need. In the mind of the medical team, however, she is making a bad decision because she is thwarting her ability to live and prolong life. Medical teams sometimes try to persuade Jehovah's Witness patients to allow blood transfusions—or, what is more problematical, transfuse them if they are comatose. Ethical patient care requires that the medical team realize that fulfilling spiritual needs is more important than fulfilling physiological needs because spiritual needs have the most important place in the levels of human needs.

To facilitate ethical decision making, ethical norms have been constructed that express which actions are good and which are bad. These ethical norms are an effort to codify or express the experience that people have had when making individual ethical decisions. Therefore, we have positive ethical norms, such as "tell the truth" and "honor your father and mother," and negative ethical norms, such as "do not steal" and "do not commit adultery." In most cases, these norms can simply be followed without a great deal of discussion because usually their validity can be easily discerned. Sometimes, however, more investigation is needed to see if the norm has validity for a particular action—that is, whether the particular act in question corresponds to the norm. Thus, the good protected by observing the ethical norm "do not steal" is the good of private property. Could it happen that a person would starve to death if she did not steal some money or food? Is the good of human life more important than the good of private property? Thus, some ethical norms are subject to evaluation when it seems the norm would impose irrational behavior. The circumstances in which acts are performed may change the ethical evaluation of the act. Is this analysis true of all ethical norms? Are all ethical norms relative in the sense that circumstances may change the authority of the norm? This issue is highly debated in ethics. As the essays in this volume illustrate, some ethical norms—such as respecting the worth of innocent human life—are so important that they oblige under all conditions and circumstances. At times, however, the circumstances of an act will have a greater impact on the morality of the act. For example, determining whether the removal of life support is ethical or unethical depends on the circumstances that relate to the patient's medical condition. Given the medical condition of the patient, will continued use of a respirator be beneficial for the patient? As we shall see in some of the essays contained in this book, the meaning of the word "benefit" is open to different interpretations.

In the course of history, several general norms have been formulated to guide the ethical practice of medicine. These norms are derived from the experience of physicians and nurses seeking to fulfill the needs of patients and caregivers in a balanced manner. Because ethical medicine seeks to fulfill all the needs of the patient, an ethical physician or nurse seeks to do more than keep the patient alive. Some of the norms for the ethical practice of medicine are the following:

1. Do no harm to the patient.
2. Obtain informed consent from the patient or the patient's proxy.
3. Respect human life and bodily integrity.
4. Tell the truth.
5. Maintain confidentiality, especially concerning harmful facts and information.
6. Respect the spiritual path of the patient.
7. Do not use patients in research projects without their consent.
8. Allow patients to die if life-prolonging therapy is ineffective or imposes an excessive burden.
9. Offer health care because people are in need, not because they can pay for it.

Clearly, in applying these norms, there is often a need to resolve conflicts that arise between different norms. For example, do community needs ever modify the norm to observe confidentiality? It seems so, because cases of venereal disease must be reported to public authorities so the community may take steps to limit the disease. More concretely, how far can we go in observing norm 9 without impeding the effort to provide health care for those who are able to pay for their care? Most of the time, however, these principles can be applied correctly with little discussion about their meaning or applicability.

Taking time to study carefully whether a particular action will fulfill the human needs of a particular person in a balanced manner is a time-consuming and difficult process. For this reason, when we make ethical decisions in health care, we must know the medical facts; that is, we must ascertain the diagnosis and prognosis. Often the diagnosis and prognosis will not be certain; thus, uncertainty is often a factor that makes ethical decisions in health care confusing or difficult. With regard to removing life support, for example, the ethical decision is often made more difficult because the effect of removing the life support is often unknown: Will continuing the life support be a benefit for the patient, or will it be ineffective or an excessive burden? If some degree of moral certitude cannot be obtained, sound ethical decision making requires that the more cautious action—the action most likely to protect patient benefit—should be followed. After discerning the medical facts, we must analyze the options for action insofar as patient benefit is concerned. These options must be compared with one another. Unfortunately, perfect options are seldom available.

Given the circumstances, the best or better option must be selected. Often the choice of the better or best option will result from a comparison of human needs that will be fulfilled by the particular options. Patient bene-fit must take into consideration the four basic levels of human needs men-tioned earlier. Ultimately, one option must be selected. Theoretically, the option chosen will not always be the perfect option, objectively speaking, but it should be an option substantiated by moral certitude as the best option under the present circumstances. If a list of options for treating some illnesses are suggested, one may be too expensive or impose excessive bur-dens. For example, the best treatment for emphysema may be to move to a warm and dry climate. Not many people have the money to relocate or the inclination to leave friends and family, however. Thus, an option for treat-ing the emphysema must be chosen that in theory is less effective but is the best hope for cure or palliative care under the circumstances.

Given what is known at this time, and given what we can predict about the future, acting in this way seems to be the best manner to promote the well-being of the patient. This process of decision making is called reasoned analysis or personalism because it endeavors to bring human reason to the center of ethical decision making and seeks to benefit persons in their quest for human fulfillment.[1]

Sometimes the process of reasoned analysis may be shortened through the use of moral norms, but, as explained above, the moral norms them-selves will be the subject of reasoned analysis in some particular situations. Because the process of evaluating human needs and determining whether an action fulfills those needs in a balanced manner through reasoned analysis is time-consuming and difficult, there is a tendency among human beings to make ethical decisions through other methods. We offer a brief description of some of these methods and point out the shortcomings of these methods in chapter 2. In one way or another, these methods dispose for ethical error because they do not utilize a thorough analysis of the four human needs as an integral part of the process of decision making.

Conclusions

In conclusion, let us consider a description of the collaborative process of reasoned analysis for making ethical decisions in regard to matters of health care.

1. Discern important medical facts affecting the basic needs of the patient.
2. Discern conflicts in fulfilling needs; if there are no conflicts, there probably is no ethical problem.

3. Consider the various options for fulfilling patient's needs. If a conflict arises in regard to patient need, consult the patient or proxy.

4. Following the moral principle of informed consent, determine with the patient or proxy which option, here and now, will best fulfill the patient's need in an integrated manner. Ethical principles will usually help in this step of process.

5. If you are morally certain that the option selected is a good ethical decision, follow through with it. If you have serious doubts, confirm your choice by comparing it to other cases and discussing it with others.

Note

1. Benedict Ashley and Kevin O'Rourke, *Health Care Ethics: A Theological Analysis,* 4th ed. (Washington, D.C.: Georgetown University Press, 1997). Chapter 7.

Chapter 2 _____

Other Ethical Systems

Why do different people arrive at different solutions to ethical problems in medicine even if they begin with the same set of facts? Why, for example, do some persons—whether physicians or family members—decide it is an act of mercy to remove artificial nutrition and hydration from a patient in an irreversible coma, whereas others would maintain that the same action would be murder? One reason for disparate ethical decisions is because people use different ethical systems in reaching decisions about right and wrong actions. In this chapter we describe briefly the various systems that people use to reach ethical decisions. Then we evaluate these systems according to their effectiveness in a pluralistic society.

Ethics seeks to determine which actions will contribute to a person's fulfillment or happiness. Ethics presupposes human freedom and human responsibility. When judging which actions to perform—such as whether to gain money by stealing or through work—a person often faces a conflict. One action is good from one point of view: Stealing is often an easier and quicker way of obtaining money. The other action, however, is good from another point of view: Working enables one to retain personal integrity, respect the rights of others, and avoid the disgrace associated with theft. How do people settle the conflict? Whether they realize it or not, people use a consistent method of ethical decision making when they are faced with such questions. The major systems of ethical decision making are:

1. *Emotivism.* This ethical theory relies mainly on subjective, emotional response. According to this theory, something is right or wrong because "I feel it is right or wrong." In the United States today, this method of ethical reasoning is widespread. Many people will defend their own or others' ethical choices as long as the people making decisions are "sincere." This method of decision making leads to exaggerated individualism, as Robert Bellah and others demonstrate in *Habits of the Heart.*[1] Although emotions are an important factor in making good ethical decisions, emotions alone do not offer a sufficient basis for developing a system of shared values in a pluralistic society. Moreover, emotivism does not enable one to measure an action in accord with one's human fulfillment, unless one maintains that emotional satisfaction is the same as human fulfillment.

2. *Legalism.* This ethical system maintains that the law, whether rendered in statutes or court decisions, determines what is ethical. In health care this method is often used with a view toward avoiding malpractice litigation. Thus, physicians, hospital administrators, trustees, and their legal advisers often ask, "What will help us avoid malpractice?" rather than, "How do we foster patient benefit?" This method perverts the relationship between ethics and law. Laws should be founded on ethical norms but the law often falls behind ethical thinking. For example, to assert that artificial hydration or feeding cannot be removed unless there is a law enabling people to do so ignores the essential goal of medical care. Thus, laws are helpful if they express sound ethical norms, but laws are not the ultimate norm for ethical choices in a pluralistic society. Too often, laws and

court decisions are based merely on legal precedent or political expediency. Thus, they are not always a reliable guide for ethical decision making.

3. *Cultural Relativism.* This ethical method decrees that actions are ethical if they correspond to the customs of a society or a segment of society. Simply because people are accustomed to performing actions, however, does not mean that this custom is an ultimate judge of these actions' ethical worth. Probably the most significant examples of cultural relativism for the health care professions are found in the various codes of ethics used by different associations. For example, the American Medical Association's Code of Ethics approves of some actions that are in themselves unethical and disapproves of others that are not unethical (for example, performing fetal research, abortions, and facilitating surrogate motherhood). However, no substantial reasons are given for the decisions offered. Does one have to follow the codes in question to be a good physician? In the past, the codes of ethics for physicians have contained blatant violations of patients' rights, especially with regard to informed consent.[2] Thus, customs and codes are only worthwhile if they are subject to more basic ethical evaluation. An action is not ethical in our pluralistic society simply because "everyone does it."

4. *Fideism.* This method of ethical decision making is based on religious faith in a church or a person. Although church directives may be helpful and fulfilling for human beings, and many churches offer worthwhile and reasonable explanations for their teachings, the ultimate motivation for accepting the teaching is religious faith. Thus, the directives of churches, even though reasonable, will not be accepted in a pluralistic society by people who do not share the same faith.

5. *Reasoned Analysis.* This method judges ethical issues by reasoning about the effect of the action on important values of life and the consequences of the action on persons involved (see chapter 1). This system seeks to discern whether the action and its consequences contribute to human fulfillment and happiness. Reasoned analysis in ethical investigation is difficult and intricate because it means one must seek some common definitions pertinent to human fulfillment and happiness. It also means that one must formulate general norms concerning human functions and human values and be ready to follow these general norms.

Reasoned analysis in ethical decision making is complicated and intricate, but it has been successful in the health care field because many norms have been accepted with regard to ethical health care. For example, all ethicists accept that medical personnel should obtain informed consent before treating patients because this disposes for human fulfillment. Likewise, most accept that access to health care for poor people is a public concern. The many volumes published by the President's Commission for the Study of Ethical Problems in Medicine and Biomedical and Behavioral Research are examples of the effort to approach ethics through reasoned analysis.

Although agreement exists on many major ethical issues in medicine, we do not mean to imply that all ethical issues are near solution. The ethical evaluation of abortion is one area in which consensus has not materialized. We do insist, however, that reaching consensus on abortion and other complicated ethical issues in our pluralistic society is not possible unless a process of patient and comprehensive examination of the ethical issues occurs through reasoned analysis. Only through this method can consensus be developed concerning actions that foster or impede human development. Only then will we have the opportunity for consensus in our pluralistic society.

Conclusion

Many books describe in detail the various ethical systems. This brief synopsis presents a general idea of each system and why we often differ on ethical conclusions even though we may begin with the same set of facts.

The next time you seek to make an ethical judgment or are involved in an ethical debate, analyze the method of decision making that you are using. Realize that some methods are not well founded because they do not ask basic questions. Also, realize or recall that our pluralistic society needs a method of ethical decision making that is founded on reasoned analysis of shared values.

Notes

1. Robert Bellah et al., *Habits of the Heart* (New York: Harper & Row, 1985).
2. Carleton B. Chapman, *Physicians, Law, and Ethics* (New York: New York University Press, 1984).

Chapter 3 _____

Medical Ethics Needs Accurate Distinctions

A few years ago, Larry McAfee, a young man in Georgia who is a quadriplegic and permanently dependent upon a ventilator, wished to remove the ventilator because in his judgment it resulted in more burden than benefit. Because death would result indirectly as a result of removing the ventilator, he and his family were forced to go to court to gain legal approval for the proposed removal. In reporting the decision of Judge Edward Johnson, one newspaper headline stated, "Judge Gives Quadriplegic Permission to Commit Suicide"; another stated, "Judge Rules Quad Free To End His Own Life." The reporting of this case reminds us of the importance of making accurate distinctions when making an ethical analysis. Indeed, much of the disagreement and misunderstanding with regard to ethical decisions often seems to stem from a lack of clear distinctions. This chapter analyzes some ethical terms that often generate confusion because they may be used with different meanings.

Terminal Illness. This term may signify that a patient will die in the immediate future even if life-support therapy is used; for example, a patient with cancer in several vital organs will die soon, no matter what therapy is employed. Terminal illness may also indicate the presence of a fatal pathology that will cause death in the immediate future *unless* therapy or life support is used. For example, a person with renal failure has a terminal illness in this sense, but life may be prolonged through dialysis or a kidney transplant. Many people believe that a decision to withhold life support may be made only when a terminal illness is present in the first meaning of this term—that is, when the therapy is useless. Catholic teaching allows therapy to be withheld when the second meaning of the term is verified and the therapy would result in a grave burden for the patient. Judge Johnson used this meaning of "terminal illness" in the McAfee case.

Quality of Life. This term is sometimes used in situations in which a physical or mental disability impairs a person's function but does not endanger the person's life. For example, a crippled person confined to a bed might be said to have a low quality of life if the term is used with this meaning. The term can also be used, however, to refer to a person whose ability to function is seriously impaired as a result of a serious pathology *and whose life is endangered* as a result of the pathology—for example, a person who is neurologically impaired because of advanced cancer of the central nervous system.

The confusion arising from the use of this term without proper distinction is monumental. Some people believe that life support should never be withdrawn for "quality of life" reasons. This judgment is true if "quality of life" is used in the first sense. It is not true, however, if "quality of life" is used in the second sense. Indeed, even people who denounce "quality of life" as a criterion for removing life support will admit that life support can be withdrawn if the condition of the patient is hopeless. This admission acknowledges that "quality of life" in the second sense may be used as a reason for removing life support. To avoid confusion arising from use of this term, Thomas O'Donnell, S.J., introduced the term "quality of function" and suggests that it be substituted when "quality of life" is used in the second sense. This substitution seems to obviate the confusion arising from the unspecified use of "quality of life."

Active and Passive Euthanasia. Through this distinction, people sometimes convey the notion that active euthanasia (inducing a cause of death) is morally wrong, but passive euthanasia (withholding care with the intention of letting a person die) is morally acceptable. The intention of killing a person either by inducing the cause of death or by being passive and allowing death to occur is ethically unacceptable, however. Withholding or removing life support from a person is ethically acceptable only if life support will not benefit the patient and the intention of the caregiver is to do something morally good—that is, to cease doing something useless or to avoid inflicting a grave burden on the patient. As Pope Pius XII pointed out, removing life support with the intention of benefiting the patient even if death is foreseen is an application of the principle of double effect (or indirect voluntary effect).[1]

Ordinary and Extraordinary Means to Prolong Life. Although people sometimes use this term as though its meaning were self-evident, this term has medical and ethical connotations. From a medical perspective, a therapy is ordinary if it is standard or accepted; for example, clearing the air passages of a newborn infant is ordinary care, medically speaking. From the medical perspective, a means to prolong life is extraordinary if it is innovative, unusual, or unproven; for example, gene splicing to cure thalassemia is extraordinary medical care. From an ethical perspective, however, ordinary care signifies medical care that is morally obligatory because it is effective and does not impose a grave burden. Extraordinary care is morally optional because its use is ineffective or does impose a grave burden. From a medical perspective, a therapy or life-support device can be judged ordinary or extraordinary before it is utilized for a particular patient. From the ethical perspective, however, these terms may not be applied unless the medical condition of the patient is known. Moreover, from the ethical perspective a therapy or life-prolonging mechanism may be judged acceptable by one person with a low quality of function but too burdensome by another person with the same low quality of function. Not every quadriplegic would make the same decision as Larry McAfee because not every person would judge the use of the ventilator to be a grave burden. Indeed, after encouragement offered by other people with disabilities, Larry McAfee changed his mind about removing the ventilator and is still alive today.

When analyzing the burden resulting from therapy, some people consider only the physiological effects of the therapy or consider the therapy as though it had ethical import apart from the person to whom it will be applied. Thus, some people hold up a gastrostomy tube and a can of Ensure at national meetings and state, "Installing this tube and administering nutrition through the tube would never be a grave burden because this tube and Ensure are not expensive, and tube feeding does not inflict serious pain." Catholic teaching with regard to grave burden, however, maintains that the burden from therapy may affect the psychological, social, and spiritual functions of the person as well as the physiological. Moreover, assessing the burden of a therapy apart from the wishes of the person to whom it will be applied is the same as buying a suit without knowing the correct size or color preference. Finally, some people would confine assessment of burden only to the very act utilizing the therapy. As John Connery, S.J., pointed out, however, when considering the history of Catholic teaching in regard to grave burden, "In assessing any particular means, it made no difference whether the burden to the patient was experienced before, during, or after the treatment."[2]

Conclusion

The analysis of the foregoing terms is not intended to answer any specific ethical questions. The potential ambiguity of these terms, however, indicates the need for clarification of terms before specific ethical judgments are offered.

Notes

1. Pope Pius XII. "The Prolongation of Life" (November 24, 1957), in *Issues in Ethical Decision Making,* ed. Gary Atkinson (St. Louis: Pope John XXIII Center, 1976).
2. "Prolonging Life: The Duty and Its Limits," *Catholic Mind* (October 1980), 45.

Chapter 4

The Values Inherent in Medical Care

Values influence—and in many cases determine—human behavior; they give direction and meaning not only to individual actions but also to our personalities. What values are associated with health care? Are any values so closely associated with medical care that neglecting them would frustrate the effort to offer that care? To study these questions adequately, we shall consider the concepts of health, human function, and health care.

Principles

Health and health care are interdependent. Hence, to understand the values associated with health care, one must possess a clear notion of human health. Ask the physician, nurse, or hospital administrator, "What is health?" and you are liable to receive a blank look in reply. Henrik Blum concludes a searching analysis of the concept of health with the brief formula, "Health is the state of being in which an individual does the best with the capacities he has, and acts in ways that maximize his system."[1] Because a human being is an organism, it is an open system. Hence, in maintaining balance or homeostasis, a person is continually relating to the environment.

For our purposes, then, we conceive of health as optimal human functioning, which implies not only internal harmony and consistency of function, but the capacity of the organism to maintain itself in its environment.

What does the term "human function" convey? Human beings are born with the need to eat—because we feel hunger (the need for nutrition in order to survive), we perform the function of eating. We have a capacity for knowledge—because we feel a need for truth in order to understand and fulfill our purpose in life, we perform the function of learning. Ethicists widely acknowledge that there are four categories of human needs and corresponding functions: (1) biological or physiological; (2) psychological; (3) social; and (4) spiritual or creative.

Given these basic needs and functions, it is extremely important to discern how they are related because this relationship will provide a blueprint for the quest for health and the limits of medical care. Is one function more important than another? If so, it will contribute more to health. Are the relationships among the various functions cooperative or competitive? Can one function be sacrificed for another without impairing the individual's health?

These four functions are not stories in a building, one on top of the other, but interrelated dimensions of human activity. Just as the length, height, and depth of a cube can be distinguished conceptually for the sake of study but not separated in reality, the four basic human functions are interconnected. Every truly human act involves all four functions. A human spiritual act, whether it is the creative act of a scientist or the loving act of a parent, involves a biological, psychological, and social function at the same time. Although one type of function will predominate in a human act, all types will be present.

The task of the creative function is to integrate the biological, psychological, and social functions. Thus, creative functions are the deepest, most central, and most complex. At the same time, however, these activities are rooted in and dependent on the other functions in a network of interrelations. One cannot think unless one's brain is physiologically sound. Even though these function are interdependent, each function is to a certain extent independent—structurally and functionally differentiated—so that when help in restoring function is needed, each function is served by a different discipline. To restore the physiological function of bone structure, for instance, an orthopedist is called; for psychological function, a psychologist or psychiatrist is needed; for the social function, a social counselor or lawyer is required; for the creative-spiritual function, a teacher or spiritual director is called for.

The ultimate goal of health care, then, is an optimally functioning human person. This concept is richer and more complex than the ultimate goal put forward for health care by many ethicists: the autonomy of the person.[2]

Discussion

Clearly, physicians and all other medical care professionals must be concerned proximately and primarily with healing the physiological and psychological functions. Their efforts at restoring these functions must be performed, however, with the awareness of the interrelatedness of all human functions. Thus, the ultimate goal of health care must be health in the fuller sense: the coordinated functioning of all human powers. Physicians who do not realize the interrelatedness of all human functions might think they have the right to make all decisions for the patient; health planning might be directed only to the betterment of physiological functions without regard for their relation to psychological, social, or spiritual functions.

Even though patients present themselves in a wounded state of health—as a result of which they have lost some degree of self-determination—the patient's power to make his or her own decisions must be respected by the physician and all other persons in health care. Because of the good in question and because there is a need to respect the patient's spiritual integrity, a specific type of relationship arises between the physician and the patient, known familiarly as the professional relationship. The heart of this relationship is an avowal (*professio*) that one person is willing to help another person attain an important human good while respecting that person's personal worth and dignity. Given the service value in the relationship between the professional and the person in need of help, the relationship must be built on trust. This trust is especially important in medicine because the patient's vulnerability is multidimensional and the patient-physician relationship is intrinsically imbalanced.

If this brief account of the values inherent in the medical relationship is accurate, profit cannot be the primary basis of any profession but must be considered a secondary and highly variable feature. Traditionally, a principle fundamental to all professions has been that the professional must be ready to give services free to those who are in need but cannot pay. Indeed, official codes of medical ethics usually state that fees should be adjusted to the ability of the patient to pay.

In view of the foregoing discussion, the following value statements are normative for individuals and corporations involved in health care:

1. Persons offering medical care must remember and respect the worth and higher functions of the individual; this implies something more than mere "autonomy."
2. The overriding purpose of medical care must be a desire to serve persons whose physiological or psychological health is impaired to enable them to lead a better life.
3. The patient-physician relationship must be permeated by trust.
4. Medical care should not be considered a commodity—something to be bought or sold in a market system—because it is a precious and vital good to which no price can be attached and because it is pre-requisite to the attainment of other human goods as well as the pursuit of a meaningful life.

Notes

1. Henrik Blum, *Expanding Health Care Horizons: From General Systems Concept of Health Care to a National Policy* (Oakland, Third Party Publications, 1983), 27.
2. Charles J. Dougherty, *Ideal Fact and Medicine* (New York: University Press of America, 1985), 66ff.

Chapter 5 _____

Medical Ethics: Basic Goals

Many individuals and professional organizations maintain that ethics committees must be formed in hospitals to help answer questions arising from advanced technology and increased recognition of patients' rights. Even if these committees are confined to educational activities and not given the power to make ethical decisions for others, a practical question arises: What principles will the committee use in deliberating about ethical issues or trying to formulate policy to be presented to the administration for approval? Drawing together ten people with ten different ethical perspectives might bring chaos rather than consensus. Is there a common understanding of medical ethics that will enable people on ethics committees to function cooperatively and intelligently despite different professions, backgrounds, and religious persuasions?

Principles

Medical ethics arises from the relationship between a patient and a physician. The patient goes to a physician seeking health. Health, in this limited sense, is the well-being of physiological and psychological functions. Health is of great value for the patient but it is not the only value; the patient has values associated with social or spiritual functions as well.

The physician enters the relationship promising to help the patient achieve health. This promise is based on two assumptions:

1. The physician strives for competency in the field of medicine.
2. The physician promises to respect the patient as a person.

Hence, in addition to the value of health in a limited sense, the social and spiritual values the patient might have will be respected. Thus, the physician agrees to respect the patient's quest for health in the wider sense of the term. This respect for social and spiritual aspects arises from the fact that the physician respects the patient as an equal. Although the patient is subordinate or unequal to the physician in medical skill and knowledge, he or she deserves respect as a person of equal worth insofar as the other values of life are concerned.

Often there will be no conflict between the patient's health values and his or her social and spiritual values. In most circumstances, patients regard healing (a physiological or psychological value) as a necessary means for achieving other values in life (social and spiritual). Thus, in most cases, difficult ethical decisions will not be in question because no choice between conflicting values is necessary. Rather, these routine cases call only for protection of the patient's basic rights as a human being (e.g., the right to be informed, the right to maintain one's reputation).

In some cases, however, there will be a conflict between maintaining or restoring health (achieving psychological or physiological values) and achieving social or spiritual values. For example, an aging patient suffering from a terminal illness may decide that he or she would be better off spiritually if life-prolonging therapy were withdrawn and death allowed to ensue. A person who is a Jehovah's Witness might believe that divine law prohibits the use of blood transfusions even if they would prolong life. In cases of this nature, the conflict must be settled by treatment that respects the patient's values. The ethical basis for the patient's right to choose the type of treatment is the fact that as a human being the patient is equal to the physician. A patient entering the healing relationship does not surrender personal responsibility for determining which values are more important in a given situation.

Similarly, the physician does not surrender his or her value system when entering the healing relationship. Thus, physicians may have difficult ethical decisions to make as well: For example, is it contrary to my value system to allow a patient to die when I know life could be prolonged? Should I operate on the person who refuses blood transfusion knowing there is increased danger of death? The medical relationship seeks to achieve health but does not posit health as the ultimate human value for the patient or the physician.

Discussion

The goal of healing the patient in accord with his or her value system serves as the touchstone of ethical medical practice in particular and health care in general. Of course, other factors should be considered in medical and health care; for example, economic and societal factors enter into the offering of medical and health care. These economic and social factors are especially prominent today with the national focus on cost-effectiveness, competition, and reducing the use of health care facilities. Although these economic and social factors must be considered by the ethical physician or hospital administrator, they should not be allowed to dominate the practice of medical care or health care. If they do, a perversion of values occurs, and physicians and other health care professionals betray the trust of patients and their own integrity. Resisting the pressure to make economic or societal factors the basis for decision making will be difficult for ethics committees as well as for physicians and other health care professionals.

From the nature of the healing relationship and the presuppositions noted above, the general principle of medical ethics can be deduced. For example, informed consent is required to enable patients to express their value systems and ensure that they are treated as equals. Informed consent gives rise to the principle that health care professionals should tell the truth; because the patient's reputation is of great value, the principle of confidentiality is posited.

Although these and other principles of medical ethics are deduced from the nature of the physician-patient relationship, they should not be applied as though they were straitjackets determining every particular decision. In practice, two patients may be treated differently because each might have a different value system. Thus, medical ethics is not relativistic or circumstantial in that it does have valid general principles. Yet it is flexible because these general principles must be applied to individual patients who have different needs and value systems. Facing a choice between death and severely debilitated survival, one person might choose life-prolonging therapy; another might choose only pain-relieving therapy.

Conclusion

Ethics committees can be helpful if the people serving on them have a common understanding of the nature of medical ethics. Judging from the literature on the subject, however, ethics committees often seem to be promoted as a means of defusing moral responsibility, of avoiding malpractice litigation, or of removing the anguish from difficult ethical decisions. There is no way to make difficult ethical decisions easy. People serving on ethics committees would do well to ponder constantly the question: Do we have a common understanding of medical ethics?

Chapter 6 _____

Medicine: Not an Exact Science

Across the United States, people seek compensation for injuries suffered in the course of medical care. In an effort to control medical insurance rates, limit the size of awards from injuries, and improve the quality of medical practice, California and other states have revised laws regarding damages resulting from medical care and certification of physicians. Although some action is needed to limit the extent of the "malpractice mess," many of the solutions apparently are based on a false notion of medicine and health care. To provide some light in this heated discussion, a more accurate notion of medicine and medical judgments seems necessary.

Principles

Medicine is not an exact science. An exact science is a body of knowledge that allows one to reach certain conclusions from causes and to apply that knowledge without fear of error. Mathematics is an exact science. Only human error causes defects in mathematical conclusions. Although medicine applies exact sciences—for example, it relies on the sciences of anatomy, biochemistry, and pharmacology—medicine applies knowledge gained from exact sciences to particular people. Medicine aims primarily at the well-being of individual persons. Thus, the specifying elements of all knowledge and techniques are used. Medicine is relativized because of this orientation.

Moreover, medicine is concerned with preventing and curing illness. In both cases, medicine cannot formulate specific norms that are certain to apply for all people or express ineluctable diagnoses or prognoses. When prevention of illness or disease is in question, the potential for framing scientific norms or regulations is impossible. Some people even maintain that the "science" of preventive medicine has been so overrated as to destroy its worth.[1] Although one can improve one's well-being to some extent through regimen and discipline and perhaps limit the possibility of contracting certain diseases, no definite connection exists between lifestyle and avoiding disease. Although one may never have smoked cigarettes, one has no guarantee that one will never contract lung cancer.

With regard to curing illness, the intrinsic causes of uncertainty and error are even more prevalent and serious. First, individuals are different in their physiological makeup. Thus, medical diagnosis and prognosis are not precise and exact. Through their bodies, human beings may be studied and objectified. From this study, general scientific conclusions about health, disease, and etiological agents of disease may be drawn. However, the uniqueness of each human person, which is expressed in the individual's body, cannot be generalized and objectified. The response of each patient to therapy cannot be predicted scientifically. The "art of medicine" is operative when science is applied to the individual. Because the physician assumes responsibility to help the patient strive for health, medicine is a unique form of art because its "work" is a better human being, not merely an improved inanimate object. The uniqueness of each human body is illustrated in all therapies but most especially in the use of pharmaceutical compounds.

Although drugs are tested for adverse effects through clinical trials before their approval by the Food and Drug Administration, the search for harmful side effects after approval must continue because pharmacological compounds affect different people in different ways.[2] Penicillin, for example, serves as a forceful antimicrobial agent for most people; for some people, however, it triggers a toxic or allergic reaction that can be fatal.

A second factor limiting the certainty of medical judgments is the difficulty in obtaining sufficient empirical evidence to guarantee the certainty of the medical diagnosis. The anatomy of a clinical judgment combines inductive and deductive reasoning and is filled with uncertainties. Symptoms may be similar for several illnesses or diseases. Moreover, even if laboratory tests are used in making a diagnosis, they may vary widely in reliability and accuracy. Thus, even if tests are available and symptoms abound, the diagnosis of an illness is tentative. One conclusion may be more probable than another but far from certain because the "right" information might be unobtainable. In sum, the process of reaching a diagnosis is dialectical, not the result of rigorous scientific reasoning. The potential for misdiagnosis is evidenced by autopsy studies that show that the correlation between the cause of death and the clinical diagnosis is far from exact.

Finally, another cause for uncertainty and ambiguity in medical decision making is the value system of the patient. Medicine is primarily concerned with the patient's physiological well-being, but this well-being in turn is directed to the individual's social and spiritual (cognitive-affective) good. In other words, although physiological health is a foundational value of human life, it is not the only value. A patient may have social or spiritual values that will determine the type of medical treatment he or she chooses to receive. Thus, the "right" physiological therapy for a particular person may not always coincide with the patient's value system. The person suffering from cancer may determine to forgo curative or palliative treatment to devote his or her life savings to his or her children's education rather than to therapy that may not be successful. The importance of the patient's value system and its influence on therapeutic choices is a vital element in medical decision making. Clearly, the patient's value system is another source of uncertainty in reaching therapeutic conclusions.

Discussion

Why do people believe that physicians are able to make completely accurate diagnoses about illnesses and infallible decisions about healing therapies for various diseases? Why does the general public, especially members of juries, usually presume that "someone has to pay" if a patient suffers an injury in the course of medical care? Pellegrino and Thomasma[3] attribute this prevalent mistaken notion about medicine to Cartesian dualism. Descartes separated the person and the body, seeking mathematical certainty in medicine. As a result, however, he introduced a false dichotomy that presented the human body as a machine, an entity that could be disassembled and repaired like other machines. This concept dehumanizes medicine. One must also admit that the medical profession has not sought avidly to dispel the aura of infallibility surrounding it.

Given the intrinsic uncertainty of medical decision making, therefore, plans to evaluate physicians because of their "mistakes" are unsound. Attendance at continuing education programs may be required of physicians, but it is unjust to measure medical acumen by counting "mistakes" or malpractice accusations. Injuries resulting from patient neglect or physician impairment should be declared as such and just compensation offered. For this reason, physician review boards should be composed of consumers as well as professionals. A contract of justice exists between physician and patient, and the physician should be held to make restitution if he or she does not fulfill the object of the contract. The contract's object is not a certain scientific diagnosis or prognosis, however. Rather, this contract is a dialectical decision founded on scientific knowledge but influenced by the particular physiology of the body; the ambiguity of symptoms, signs, and tests; and the differing value systems of individual persons.

Conclusion

Applying the foregoing concepts will not eliminate all problems arising from medical practice. The perspective of the general public, legislators, judges, and juries, however, may be more accurate if they realize that medicine is not an exact science and that physicians make judgments that "follow the rules" but still may be inefficacious. In their diagnoses and prognoses, physicians may be in error through no moral, cognitive, or technological fault of their own.

Notes

1. Lenn E. Goodman and Madeleine J. Goodman, "*Prevention—How Misuse of a Concept Undercuts its Worth.*" Hastings Center Report 16, no. 2 (April 1986): 26–27.

2. Gerald Faich, "Adverse Drug-Reaction Monitoring." *New England Journal of Medicine* 314, no. 24 (June 12, 1986): 1589–92.
3. Edmund Pellegrino and David Thomasma, *A Philosophical Basis of Medical Practice* (New York: Oxford University Press, 1981), 99.

Chapter 7

Professionalism: The Essence Is Empathy

The concern for ensuring ethical behavior on the part of health care professionals continues to mount. The Federal government approved regulations that limit investments in clinics and laboratories by physicians receiving Medicare or Medicaid payments. The American Surgical Association promulgates norms to control promotional activities of members lest they receive undue compensation from medical supply or pharmaceutical companies. Prominent voices in health care are concerned about the erosion of trust that results from entrepreneurial activities of physicians and hospitals. Will the aforementioned admonitions and norms be effective? Not if they stand alone. To create an ethical atmosphere in the corporate culture of health care, a renewed emphasis on self-fulfillment through service to patients is needed. A sense of professionalism must be fostered to ensure that ethics leaves the realm of theory and becomes characteristic of everyday activities of health care professionals. In this chapter we consider the meaning of professionalism and its implications for people in health care.

Principles

Professionalism requires knowledge, skill, and empathy. The knowledge required to qualify as a professional varies depending on one's role in the provision of health care. In the past physicians were considered the

only health care professionals; in the nineteenth century nursing was recognized as a profession as well. In the twentieth century many additional
occupations and services in health care have been recognized as professions because of additional knowledge about human physiology and psychology and the skills developed to apply this knowledge. In our day,
therefore, several new professionals may be listed in the field of health
care—for example, physicians assistants, physical therapists, and health
care administrators.

Clearly, the knowledge necessary for professional practice is not acquired
"once and for all." The need to continue learning even after having attained
professional status is well recognized. Unfortunately, many health care professionals confine their continuing education to their own specialties.
Although emphasis on improving scientific knowledge is laudable, some
effort to advance one's humanistic knowledge is also useful if one is to
progress as a professional.

The skills associated with a profession are designed to utilize effectively
the knowledge proper to that profession. In the United States the effort to
acquire knowledge and skills simultaneously is highly developed in the
health care professions. All health care educational programs feature clinical experience as an integral element.

Although knowledge and skill are important for caregivers, the distinguishing characteristic of any profession is empathy—the ability "to get
inside" the patient or client. Empathy is defined as "the capacity for participation in another's feelings and ideas." Professions are distinguished from
trades, crafts, or commercial occupations by reason of the need for empathy. A tradesperson or artisan—for example, a plumber or electrician—
can perform his or her service even if he or she knows nothing about the
person who requested the service. The knowledge and skill of the plumber
or electrician ensure that a building will have water and electricity. Although
the people who utilize the building may benefit from the ready supply of
electricity and water, the person installing or repairing the electrical or
plumbing equipment need never contact the persons living there. Professionals, on the other hand, must know their clients well to accomplish
their goals. They help people strive for goods that require cognitive and
affective function on the part of the client. Professions are directed toward
helping people achieve goods that are fundamental and esteemed because
they are goods that bespeak our humanity. Health, for example, is one of
the basic goods of human life. Without health we have a difficult time performing actions that are an expression of the fullness of our humanity.
Pursuing truth or building community are two endeavors by which one

measures one's humanity. Cannot one pursue these goods more effectively if one is healthy?

Discussion

The extent to which empathy is neglected in contemporary society was evidenced in a statement by Tom Peters, coauthor of *In Search of Excellence* (the "bible" for developing effective business organizations). This book emphasizes the importance of values insofar as creating effective business organizations is concerned. Peters admits, however, that he neglected to stress the need for empathy in developing value-centered people who will develop value-centered organizations. As Peters states, "(Empathy) is a simple notion, but it is the most complex and operationally the most difficult among the principles that all successful institutions observe. There is nothing patronizing or condescending about empathy. It requires a depth of sensitivity that allows one to sense other people's needs, often before they themselves articulate them." Peters concludes, "I am still at a loss as to how to be prescriptive about empathy, but the term will never again be far from my lips."[1]

Although Peters may be hesitant about being prescriptive in this matter, a few observations about developing empathy are in order. Empathy must be based on a desire to share one's gifts with other persons. The gifts a professional possesses are knowledge and skill concerning the attainment of an important human good. Being a professional is sometimes described as an altruistic endeavor. In one sense that description is accurate; being a professional is being "for others." In another sense, however, being a professional is self-fulfilling because it enables people to "love others as they love themselves."

The second basis for developing empathy is respect, acceptance, and reverence for other people. Before one can cultivate the ability "to participate in another's feelings and ideas," one must have a recognition of the person as "another self." This concept of empathy offers an understanding of why the profession of health care brings out the best in people and why adequate health care is fundamental to developing a beneficent society.

Conclusion

Norms indicating the ethical manner to conduct oneself as a health care professional are useful. They will not be observed, however, unless individuals have a personal commitment to being professionals in the full sense of the term. Being a professional means more than earning a degree or possessing knowledge and skills. It also requires an ability "to get inside another person."

Note

1. Thomas Peters, "In Search of Excellence," *Chicago Tribune,* June 18, 1989.

Chapter 8 _____

Professional Attitudes—The Ethical Physician

Self-understanding is the beginning of wisdom but it requires the benefit of honest reactions from other people. Otherwise, no opportunity exists for objective evaluation and testing of one's subjective thoughts and attitudes.

What is true of individuals is true of a profession as well. Unless the members of a profession receive honest and objective information from people outside the profession, there is little hope for healthy and effective self-understanding. Over the past few years, the profession of medicine has received candid and worthwhile evaluations in regard to its ethical perspectives and standards from scholars outside the profession.[1] Some of these evaluations may be summarized as follows:

1. Most physicians have a strong sense of "vocation" rooted in the original priestly character of medicine and reinforced in American culture by the religious stress on vocation. Yet this religious motivation has been covered over: "The vast growth of science and technology in the 400 years since Luther has obscured the specifically religious conception of most vocations. The physician seldom speaks of God anymore when discussing his concern for the patient. Yet he still finds satisfaction in measuring up to personal standards."[2]

2. To be effective, physicians maintain that they must be motivated and competent and show concern for the patient. An important component of motivation is physicians' sense of specific competence; that is, they have an important and well-defined service to offer. Much of the personal satisfaction that physicians derive from their work depends on this sense of competence. Most physicians believe they must care for "the whole patient," but only a minority of physicians have a well-developed social conscience.

3. Physicians tend to think pragmatically; their basic attitude can be characterized as follows: "The physician sees himself as a professionally competent person who is in a social position to apply scientific knowledge and to exercise impartial control over the situation in order to achieve the rational goal of curing or helping a sick patient. The patient's part of the job is to trust the doctor and cooperate with him."[3]

4. Physicians on the whole do not regard themselves as research scientists but as applied scientists, and they do not clearly experience a dichotomy between the scientific and the humanistic or affective aspects of medicine. Their satisfactions are not theoretical but pragmatic.

5. Physicians take much satisfaction in their professional position as a mark of achievement. This sense of achievement is more important for physicians than monetary rewards, which they do not like to think of as a primary motivation. Moreover, although physicians gain some satisfaction from scientific interest in their work, they gain more satisfaction from therapeutic results. An important element of satisfaction or dissatisfaction is found in the sense of consistency between personal and professional ethics. Thus, physicians do seem to have a common sense of ethical purpose.

Discussion

Medical professionals should be aware of possible ethical biases, and medical education should strive to balance these biases if the medical profession is to make good ethical judgments.

1. On the whole, physicians continue to exhibit the dualistic balance between the scientific and humanistic. The balance is constantly imperiled, however, by the fact that physicians' scientific training is explicit, detailed, and specialized, whereas their humanistic and moral training is left largely to example and symbols transmitted to

them without explicit reflection or criticism. Physicians therefore assume that whereas science is exact, ethical discourse is vague, subjective, and a matter of opinion. On the one hand, this assumption leads to a kind of moral skepticism; on the other, it leads to a dogmatic rigidity because no method of dialogue or research for critical consensus is available.

2. Physicians tend "to take a pragmatic view whereby what is most valued is an immediate, practical solution."[4] In ethical matters this pragmatism may lead physicians to act so that they will not be made to feel guilty if an action is taken against their professional or personal standards, they will not seem inhuman toward the patient, they will not go beyond the limits of the patient to wider social problems, and they may be more concerned about the law than about ethics.

3. Because physicians' motivations are so bound up with their sense of vocation, autonomy, and competence, they resent interference in their decisions. They believe that only physicians can make medical-ethical judgments and that they can be relied on to be decent and humane in these decisions. This attitude may lead to deeply felt but simplistic attitudes toward ethical questions.[5]

4. Physicians often resent the fact that so much responsibility is laid on their shoulders. They cannot understand why a wider sociological, religious, psychological, or interrelational view should be their responsibility. Physicians believe such concerns are someone else's business.

Conclusion

These attitudes undoubtedly are the result of the medical professional's need for a clear motivation, manageable responsibilities, and sufficient freedom for action and personal judgment. If these needs result in a closed attitude that renders the physician incapable of learning from others or sharing in a team effort to improve the ethical treatment of health problems on a social scale, however, they are harmful biases that may lead to gravely mistaken ethical judgment.

Notes

1. Amasa Ford, *The Doctor's Perspective: Physicians View Their Patients and Their Practice* (Cleveland: Case Western Reserve University Press, 1967), 139ff.

2. Ibid., 140.
3. Ibid., 144.
4. Eliot Freidson, *Profession of Medicine, A Study of the Sociology of Applied Knowledge* (New York: Dodd Mead, 1971), 147.
5. Wendy Carlton, *In Our Professional Opinion* (South Bend, Ind.: University of Notre Dame Press, 1979), 173.

Chapter 9 _____

Human Rights and Health Care

In discussions of social problems, the words "human rights" frequently crop up. Often, the term is used as an absolute   as a weapon designed to settle all controversy: If one person has a human right to something, others are morally obligated to do everything in their power to ensure that the person's right is fulfilled, regardless of the nature of that right. Obviously, a few distinctions are in order if the concept of human rights is to contribute to peaceful and productive human relationships. After presenting these distinctions, this chapter asks whether health care is a human right and then offers some ethical considerations pertaining to health care as a human right.

Principles

Understanding the concept of human rights begins with an understanding of the concept of innate or fundamental goods of human life. Innate or fundamental goods are goods toward which our instincts and powers are naturally directed. The term "human right," then, is correlative with innate or fundamental good. If something is an innate or fundamental good, there is a corresponding human right to pursue that good. The Declaration of Independence lists life, liberty, and the pursuit of happiness as among innate or fundamental goods. Philosophers and ethicists have formulated longer lists of fundamental goods. For convenience's sake, all fundamental goods can be reduced to these four: prolonging life, forming human communities, providing for the future of human communities through the generation and education of children, and pursuing knowledge or wisdom.

Clearly, each innate or fundamental good has other goods closely allied with it. As we seek to prolong life, we realize that food is a necessary good. As we seek to create human communities, we realize that justice is necessary. As we seek to generate and educate children, the necessity of monogamous relationships between mother and father becomes evident. As we seek to acquire knowledge and wisdom, we realize that study and reflection are necessary human goods. Hence, an analysis of fundamental human goods reveals that there are several goods that are so closely allied with the four fundamental human goods that they also are considered to be fundamental or basic goods.

Over time, a good that was not considered fundamental because it was not needed by a majority of people may become a fundamental good. For example, knowledge is a fundamental good because it is necessary for the well-being of individuals and society. Four hundred years ago most people could acquire the knowledge necessary to lead a good and fulfilled life without going to school. As society became more complex and more knowledge was needed to survive and thrive, however, society determined that knowledge could best be communicated through schooling or education. In time, education or schooling became a basic good, and society now agrees that there is a right to education for all.

Hence, the first implication of the term "human right" is that persons have a relationship toward a good that is fundamental—that is, toward a good that is essentially connected with leading a good and fulfilled life. Of course, we also use the word "right" to connote a relationship to a good that is not fundamental (for example, the right to a car or a piece of jewelry), but because these goods do not pertain essentially to human well-being, this type of right is not included in the term "human rights."

Achieving fundamental goods of life is so important for a person's well-being as an individual and as a member of community that people have an obligation to strive assiduously to achieve these goods. In addition, because we are social beings, people should be aided by other members of the community in the pursuit of these fundamental goods. The community aids individuals by preventing others from impeding them in the pursuit of these goods and by supporting people when they need help to pursue these goods.

Thus, the term "human right" implies a relationship or natural orientation to a fundamental good. It also implies

- that human beings strive to acquire these goods. The human condition dictates that we will not always be successful in our quest for these basic goods. Our evolution, history, and culture, however, bespeak a moral obligation to strive conscientiously for these goods to be a fulfilled member of society.
- that persons should not be impeded by others in their quest for fundamental goods. We are social beings, and we will always have limited resources to fulfill the basic needs of all. Justice demands that one person should not impede another person as both strive for the goods of life. For this reason, society needs laws and courts to ensure equal access to fundamental goods such as schooling and employment. Thus, the legal system is not a burden but a social necessity.
- that if one cannot strive for a fundamental good through personal efforts, the community of persons should help in this endeavor. This third implication also flows from our nature as social beings. Striving for the basic goods of life is not an "either-or" situation. Even when we exercise our personal responsibility, we often need the help of others as we strive to acquire basic goods. Though young persons may be conscientious in seeking knowledge, their success will also depend on good teachers.

Discussion

What does the foregoing analysis imply insofar as health care is concerned? Is there a human right to health care? Is health care intimately associated with leading a good and fulfilled life? If by *health care* we mean the assistance of persons and institutions in the health care professions, then health care is so closely related to the good of prolonging life that it is a fundamental good. In times past, many people could seek to prolong life without the help of physicians and nurses or health care institutions. As a result of scientific progress in the science and art of medicine, however, assistance from people and institutions representing the profession of health care is needed to enable patients to strive for health and thus to prolong life. Hence, there is a human right to health care, and state and federal governments should institute programs that protect this right.

After acknowledging a personal responsibility of people to strive for health and access to health care, we must exercise caution. Although many people are able to strive for health and health care through their own endeavors, we must not conclude that those who need help are deficient in their exercise of personal responsibility. People do not get sick because it is their own fault. Moreover, people in the United States who do not have access to health care are seldom responsible for their situation. For the most part, they are victims of an ineffective health care system. Finally, even if some people seem irresponsible with regard to health, the ethics and ethos of health care take account of human weakness. Compassion is an essential quality of the profession of health care and must not be neglected in the name of personal responsibility.

Society's obligation to prevent others from impeding the quest for health care will not require many positive programs on the part of state and federal governments. However, enabling people to pursue health will require heroic efforts. There must be an effort to control the cost of health care and an effort to provide access to health care for all. Having affirmed the right of the general population to health care and the responsibility of the state and federal government to promote programs that will improve access to health care, several questions remain: Does affirming a right to health care imply that all persons in society should receive the same health care? What is the most fair and effective way to promote funding for the provision of health care: through employee-funded insurance programs or through general taxation? Should the provision of health care allow a choice of physicians and health care facilities? Should payment for health care be based on fee for services or on capitation in a health care organization? Simply affirming that there is a human right to health care does not answer all ethical questions in regard to fulfilling the right to health care.

Conclusion

There is a human right to health care because health care is required to strive for a good and fulfilled human life. As the effort to recognize the right to health care leads to legislation on the part of state and federal governments in the coming years, the need to factor in personal responsibility will be important. Yet the need to recognize compassion as an essential factor in the provision of health care will be even more important. There is indeed a right to health care for all because it is a basic good. In making it possible for people to exercise this right and to strive for health, however, the nature of the health care profession must be respected.

Chapter 10 _____

Culture and Religion

Contemporary bioethicists, lawyers, and health care professionals in the United States readily acknowledge, accept, and promote the concepts of informed consent and truth-telling. This acknowledgment stems from the concept of patient autonomy grounded in the human dignity of the person. A recent article in the *Journal of the American Medical Assoication,* however, indicated that many Korean Americans and, to a lesser extent, Hispanic Americans believe that patients should not be told about metastatic cancers or terminal illness.[1] In addition, they believe that the family alone should be responsible for decisions regarding the use of life-prolonging technology. In the same issue, Carrese and Rhodes describe how something as seemingly innocuous as the inquiry about advance directives (currently required by federal law) may constitute a serious cultural affront to Navajo Indians.[2] Do the requests to shield a patient from pertinent medical information represent an actualization of the patient's best interests or a blatant disregard for the fundamental good of patient autonomy?

Unfortunately, disclosure of information represents only one issue associated with multiculturalism and religious pluralism. Did the Baby K case—which involved the provision of aggressive treatment for an anencephalic infant—represent an appropriate accommodation to the mother's religious beliefs or a foolish utilization of futile therapy? Does the abhorrence of Americans to female "circumcision" (female genital mutilation) reflect an imperialistic Western bias or an appropriate response to a horrid violation of human rights? Does the common practice of obtaining a court order for blood transfusions for the child of a Jehovah's Witness illustrate the state's duty to look after the well-being of its citizens or a trampling of religious freedom? Can culture and religion be integrated into bioethical decision making in a way that respects their contributions yet still avoids the pitfall of ethical relativism?

Principles

Most people agree that respect for other people's culture is a good thing. People consider most expressions of culture as being "value neutral."

That is, people do not believe that one culture's common beliefs, values, norms, and practices are "better" than another culture's beliefs. Religious pluralism does not enjoy as great an acceptability. Nevertheless, because of the nature of human freedom and conscience, religious freedom in the West is generally accepted, with due regard for the rights of others, public order, and the common good.

Discussions about the importance of culture and religion on ethical decision making often begin with the recognition of our commonality arising from our sharing in a common nature before moving to our differences. Everyone grapples with infirmity, suffering, death, despair, certainty, freedom, and hope. This commonality of human experience and nature, which transcends culture, becomes the basis of ethical principles. An analysis of common goods and human needs has led to initiatives such as the Universal Declaration on Human Rights and the Nuremburg and Helsinki codes.

As one moves from very broad principles and norms of bioethics—such as respect for life, justice, and autonomy—to the arena of concrete decision making, however, culture and religion provide the interpretive context in which the norms are applied. This phenomenon necessarily leads to a plurality of decisions. The question arises: Are some of those concrete decisions or methods of decision making ethically better than others?

The general acceptance of culture and religion as normative for groups of people should not be interpreted as an unqualified acceptance of all beliefs and values associated with those complex realities. For example, the world of science has its own culture that governs its practitioners' behavior. Yet the current bioethical requirement of informed consent for research subjects was spawned from the unethical behavior of a subculture within the scientific community. This subculture's mantra of pragmatism resulted in a blatant disregard for human rights. Other cultural expressions or artifacts, such as slavery and Nazism, have been condemned as illegitimate precisely because they failed to promote the human agenda and infringed on fundamental human dignity. Cultural and religious beliefs and values enjoy the presumption of acceptance as legitimate manifestations of freedom. Nevertheless, such expressions are tethered to the protection of the well-being of the individual and society. Cultural values and religious beliefs that affect ethical decision making should not be accepted on face value; they must be understood and critiqued in light of their own historical development.

In health care, the ethical appropriateness of an action stems fundamentally from the purposes of medicine, the nature of the human person, and the precepts of sound reasoning. Culture and religion help to define more clearly what is in the best interests of a patient in a given situation. Patients and

health care professionals ordinarily integrate cultural and religious considerations into their decisions. In the clinical setting, family and patient approaches to decision making usually fall along the spectrum of appropriate
shared decision making. Cultural and religious views often provide an important backdrop for patients to assess the burdens and benefits of life sustain-
ing interventions. Occasions arise, however, in which culture and religion
push the envelope of ethical acceptability. This situation gives rise to some of
the more contentious cases in bioethics. In such scenarios, society must intervene on behalf of the patient because of potential harm.

Discussion

In the case of the child of a Jehovah's Witness, when absolutely necessary, the state disregards the parents' wishes and orders a transfusion. Society justifies this procedure by claiming that the child has not ratified the
religious beliefs of the parents. Underlying that justification, however, is the
presumption that the parents' religious belief in regard to transfusion is not
sufficiently reasonable. Acceptance of an adult's decision to forego a transfusion does not imply an agreement with the religious teaching but demonstrates a respect for freedom of religion.

When families demand "futile" treatment based on cultural or religious
beliefs, health care professionals display reluctance to accommodate such
requests—especially when they result in additional harm to the patient. To
comply would violate the standards of medicine. Other authorities suggest,
however, that when no harm is involved to a third party, discretion is the
better part of valor. Given the limited number of such cases and the nebulous notion of futility, some people advocate accommodation for the sake
of promoting religious liberty.

In cases involving disclosure of information to the patient, physicians
should not accede to requests by family members to exclude the patient from
the informational and decision-making loop simply because of cultural or
religious beliefs. There are two reasons for this standard. First, membership
in a particular culture or religion does not imply acceptance of all of the
beliefs of the group. An individual's adherence to specific cultural norms
depends on education, socioeconomic status, gender, and inculturation in the
larger culture. Patients may, in fact, want information. Second, human beings
are constitutively free. To exercise that autonomy properly, one must have
appropriate information to make medical decisions. Thus, health care professionals should strive to work with the family in a cooperative rather than con-
frontational manner to determine the patient's desire to be involved in the

decision-making process. Some patients may choose to waive their right to be involved in the decision. Their exercise of autonomy involves the ceding of their rights to the family. Although this situation may not be ideal, competent individuals can define beneficence for themselves in the context of their culturally and religiously mediated value system, again with due regard for society. Information should not be forced on unwilling patients. For liability reasons, one should thoroughly document such a waiver of rights.

Respecting a person's freedom may entail allowing the person to make a culturally or religiously based decision that may not coincide with what we think is in the best interests of the patient. Often, negotiation and appropriate accommodation can resolve conflicts that emerge from cultural or religious beliefs that are incongruent with those of the profession of medicine. Because stress heightens the import of cultural and religious beliefs, insensitivity to such beliefs during a patient's illness can result in noncompliance, dissatisfaction, and an adversarial relationship. Appropriate integration of cultural and religious beliefs presumes a general respect for such beliefs and an avoidance of ethnocentrism. To deal successfully with multiculturalism and religious pluralism, one must communicate effectively and ask questions to understand cultural differences. How do patients understand their illness? How does the family fit into the patient's decision making? Are there translators, ministers, and other cultural informants who can assist in dealing with patients of different cultures or religions? Is one being careful not to stereotype the patients? Given the complexity of these realities, it will take time and perseverance to resolve clinical disputes.

Conclusion

Ethical norms ultimately transcend specific cultural and religious beliefs. Such norms are specified, however, within a context that integrates culture, religion, the law, professional standards, and organizational policies. The appropriate integration of this constellation of values may stretch one's patience. By sensitive listening and accommodation (when ethically appropriate), culture and religion can rightly be integrated into health care.

Notes

1. L. Blackhall et al., "Ethnicity and Attitudes Toward Patient Autonomy," *JAMA* 274 (1995): 820–25.
2. J. Carrese and L. Rhodes, "Western Bioethics on the Navajo Reservation," *JAMA* 274 (1995): 826–29.

Chapter 11 _____

"No Greater Love"

Anyone familiar with medical ethics is aware of the principle of "double effect." The example used most frequently to illustrate this principle concerns a woman who is pregnant but also has a cancerous uterus. May the woman undergo therapy to remove or suppress the cancer, even though the infant in her womb may die as a result of the therapy? The answer to this question is in the affirmative. The woman, with the help of medical personnel, seeks a legitimate goal, namely, to prolong her life. She intends to overcome the cancer and seeks therapy. Usually surgery or chemotherapy will accomplish this goal. As a result of surgery or chemotherapy, the fetus dies. The death of the fetus is an unintended effect and therefore not morally culpable. The death of the fetus is not desired but cannot be avoided if the mother wants to overcome the cancer.

Recently, two pregnant women with cancer dramatically reversed this scenario. Both women, knowing their lives were in danger, decided to forego cancer therapy until after their babies were born. They both died shortly after giving birth. Whether they would have died within a short time even if they had undergone radiation and chemotherapy immediately is not the issue. The main issue is that their children were saved as a result of the delayed therapy.

In 1993, Barbara Barton was given two pieces of news: She was pregnant with twins, and she had chronic granulocytic leukemia. Her best chance to live, the doctors told her, was to start aggressive cancer treatment immediately, which would result in an indirect abortion of the fetuses. Mrs. Barton postponed the bone marrow transplant to protect the fetuses. Carrying the pregnancy to full term would mean she would have little chance of survival herself. A friend said, "She saw the babies as a sign. The babies meant more to her than anything." The twins were born on July 13, 1994. A few weeks later, Barbara developed a fever, indicating that her disease had worsened. Seven months later, after undergoing bone marrow therapy, she died.[1]

The case of Clemintina Geraci Winn is similar. When she was three months pregnant, doctors told her that her cancer was spreading. She could fight the cancer aggressively, causing the death of the baby, or take less hazardous drugs and carry the baby to term. She choose the latter course. By the time she gave birth, the cancer had metastasized throughout her spine, liver, and brain. Clementina spent her last days making videotapes for her son to watch as he grows up. On the tapes she told him about their Italian grandparents, about her favorite music, about her dream for him. She died March 6, 1995; her four-month-old son slept peacefully as she was buried a few days later.[2]

Principles

From an ethical perspective, both women had a choice between two goods. Either they could seek to prolong their own lives through cancer therapy, which would result in the deaths of their babies, or they could prolong the life of their babies by foregoing cancer therapy until the babies were born. Both goods—prolonging their own lives and preserving the lives of the babies—could not be accomplished simultaneously. A choice of one good over the other had to be made. The choice they made resulted in their own deaths. Was this an actual or implicit choice of suicide? Were they doing something evil to achieve a good result? To understand clearly the nature of the moral options open to the two women, let us examine more closely the moral reasoning known as the principle of double effect.

Often we choose to do something morally good that results not only in the good we intend but also in a harmful result that we do not intend. The harm results because we cannot achieve both goods at the same time. If possible, we would avoid causing the harmful result, but it is so closely entwined with the beneficial result that the beneficial result cannot be accomplished without causing the harmful result as well. Because the harmful result is beyond our true desire, it is not intended—that is, it is not freely chosen. Usually, the unwanted effect is foreseeable. Thus, the women in question knew they were shortening their own lives. To intend this result with full freedom and deliberation would be morally wrong: it would be choosing suicide. These two women were not morally responsible for shortening their lives, however, because they had no alternative once they decided to choose the good of prolonging the life of their babies.

Discussion

A clear example of double effect is depicted in the play *A Man for All Seasons* by Robert Bolt. In 1535, Sir Thomas More was commanded by King Henry VIII to swear allegiance to the King as religious head of the Catholic Church in England. If More refuses, he faces death. More has two goods he would like to preserve: his own life and allegiance to the Pope as head of the Church. Given the command of Henry VIII, however, he cannot achieve both goods. After much soul searching, More refuses to take the oath and is beheaded in the tower of London. In a way, he is responsible for his own death because he chose a good that was not compatible with prolonging his own life. Yet his own death was not something he chose directly; it was a foreseeable but indirect result of the choice of a greater good: being true to his religious faith.

The principle of double effect underlies the manner in which we are able to live with the moral decisions of everyday life. For example, many people are opposed to excessive military spending. When they pay their taxes—which they realize is a morally good action—they know that a portion of their taxes will be devoted to military spending. Should they refuse to pay their taxes if they foresee that much of the money they contribute to the common good will be used for purposes that at best are morally questionable? No, it is possible for them to express disapproval of this use for their taxes, thus making it clear that the use of tax money is beyond their direct intention when they pay their taxes. The various good causes to which their taxes will be directed are the direct intention of their effort. This is not a case of "doing more harm than good." Rather, it involves expressing a distinct division between what is intended directly and that which is forseen but not intended.

Some people object to the moral analysis of double effect, maintaining that if one knows a harmful effect will result from one's actions, one is morally responsible for that effect. This viewpoint does not appreciate the power and meaning of intention in human affairs. It is possible to be the physical cause of a result but not the moral cause of the same result. Only if the choice of the evil is direct are we morally responsible for an evil result. Opponents of this double-effect analysis of human action often neglect to speak about the good that is truly intended and to which the harmful effect is inextricably connected. Moreover, they do not differentiate between being a physical cause of a particular result and being a moral cause of a result.

Reflecting on the actions of Barbara Barton and Clementina Winn, we are struck by the generosity of these two women and the depth of love that motherhood engenders. In our materialistic world, where "everything has a price," it is edifying to reflect on the depth of a mother's love. Each person has a strong natural desire to prolong life. The love of these mothers for their children, however, led them to sacrifice their own good for the good of their children. What motivated each mother to determine that prolonging the life of her child was a greater good than prolonging her own life? Reading the accounts of their last days, it seems that neither woman ever "explained" her actions. Thus, there was no rigid logical reasoning process that led either one to forego aggressive cancer therapy to protect the life of the babies. Clementina's husband, David Winn, said he expected nothing else from his wife, "She did it because it was the right thing for her to do." As Barbara Barton died, a friend stated, "She was very matter-of-fact and didn't shed a single tear." The best decisions arise not only from a reasoned analysis of what is "right" in the ethical sense but also from a love of the good. When Thomas More's daughter declared that it would be unreasonable for him to be witness to the truth if it would result in his death, he replies, "Finally Meg, it's not a matter of reason; finally, it's a matter of love."[3]

Notes

1. "A Mother Sacrifices Life so Twins Can be Born," *New York Times,* February 9, 1995.
2. "Cancer Fells Woman Who Saved Son," *Washington Post,* March 14, 1995.
3. Robert Bolt, *A Man For All Seasons,* (New York: Vintage Books, a division of Random House), 1962.

Part Two

Informed Consent: Personal and Proxy

Chapter 12 _____

Informed Consent

Informed consent is never out of the news. Despite the emphasis given to this component of ethical medical care, difficulties in obtaining informed consent have been expressed over the years. For example, a few years ago, one author stated:

> Within one day of signing consent forms for chemotherapy, radiation therapy, or surgery, 200 cancer patients completed a test of their recall of the material in the consent explanation and filled out a questionnaire regarding their opinions of its purpose, content, and implications. Only 60 percent understood the purpose and nature of the procedure, and only 55 percent correctly listed even one major risk or complication . . . only 40 percent had read the form carefully . . . and only 27 percent could name one alternative treatment.[1]

Often the problem is the consent forms themselves. A study of consent forms from five representative hospitals revealed that the readability of all five was approximately equivalent to that of material intended for upper-division undergraduates or graduate students. Four of the five forms were written at the level of a scientific journal; the fifth was written at the level of a specialized academic magazine.

Our purpose is not to confirm or to deny the conclusions in these studies; they speak for themselves. They also offer, however, an opportunity to review some thoughts about informed consent and to discuss why it is necessary for ethical decision making.

Principles

The ethical and legal requirements for informed consent are information, comprehension, and freedom.

The specific information that should be provided for the patient concerns the purpose of the procedure, anticipated risks and benefits, alternative procedures, and hoped-for results. Information should never be withheld for the purpose of eliciting consent, and truthful answers should always be given to direct questions. If a research project is in question, certain information may be withheld provided the subject is informed that some information will not be revealed until the research is completed and that no direct harm results from withholding the information.

Comprehension of the conveyed knowledge is a more complex requirement than it might seem at first. Because subjects' capability to understand varies so greatly, the material must be adapted to the subjects' capacities. Health care professionals are responsible for ascertaining that the subject has comprehended the information, especially if the risk is serious. If the patient cannot comprehend, a third party—usually a family member but sometimes a person appointed by a court—should be asked to act in the patient's best interest. Some people have maintained that comprehension of difficult medical terms is not possible for the ordinary person, but research has shown that persons who are unfamiliar with medical terms can understand and retain explanations about medical procedures if the explanations are well-planned and stated in plain language.

Freedom implies that the person understands the situation clearly and that no coercion or undue influence is exercised by the health care professional. It is often difficult to determine, however, where justifiable persuasion ends and undue influence begins. The health care professional who believes that a particular treatment is better for the patient should state his or her conviction but should also explain clearly the reason for this opinion. Voluntariness does not imply that the patient will be free from all pressure or persuasion in a given circumstance. For example, a person with an inflamed appendix is limited insofar as freedom of choice is concerned. Voluntariness does imply that, over and above the limitations arising from the circumstances, no external coercion or moral manipulation is present.

Discussion

Some people think that informed consent is required only for research protocols or for experimental procedures. Actually, informed consent is required for any action that would affect a person's physiological, psychological, or moral integrity. Why is informed consent so important? Does it merely help avoid malpractice, or does it fulfill an important human need?

Respect for persons—one of the most basic ethical principles—is carried out in practice through informed consent. The patient's right to informed consent arises from the conviction that human beings are responsible for their own actions and their own destinies. They must be treated as equals and allowed to make the important decisions of life for themselves whenever possible. Only in this way will they be able to reach their full potential as human beings. Although the health care professional offers help to the patient, the health care professional is not given the right to make decisions for the patient, nor to manipulate the patient. Health care professionals will assist in the total and integrative betterment of the human beings they serve only if they are careful in observing the requirements of informed consent.

Note

1. B. Cassileth, "Informed Consent—Why Are Its Goals Imperfectly Realized?" *New England Journal of Medicine* 302 (1980): 896; T. Grunder, "On Readability of Surgical Consent Forms," *New England Journal of Medicine* 302 (1980): 900.

Chapter 13 _____

Proxy Consent: Deciding for Others

Four well-publicized and highly controversial legal decisions determining medical treatment for people no longer able to decide for themselves (Quinlan, Saikewicz, Spring, and Fox) call attention to the meaning of proxy consent. These cases provide a framework for reviewing the ethical norms for this type of consent and commenting briefly on the aforementioned decisions.

Whenever possible, informed consent on the part of the subject is ethically and legally necessary for every medical treatment and research project. Sometimes, however, the subject is not able to give informed consent. For example, an aged person in a coma, an infant, or a fetus cannot perform the rational act necessary for informed consent even though he or she may require some medical treatment. In such cases, another person is called on to offer informed consent; this form of consent is called proxy or vicarious consent.

Principles

Although proxy consent is often identified with personal informed consent, the two are quite different. Informed consent by a proxy is not a subspecies of personal informed consent; it is a substitute for personal informed consent and is sought when acquiring personal informed consent is impossible. For the ethical and legal use of proxy informed consent, two conditions must be present: The patient or research subject cannot offer informed consent, and the person offering the proxy consent must determine what the incompetent person would have decided if he or she were able to make the ethical decision. The second condition is difficult to ascertain and may be subject to dispute.

Decisions of proxy consent should be made in view of the good of the individual patient, not the higher good of society or a class good; the latter would amount to manipulation of the person. When deciding on treatment for a comatose person dying of cancer, for example, the proxy must seek to determine what the patient would decide if the patient were able to make the decision. Choices that would benefit people other than the patient should not be considered unless the proxy can reasonably assume that those choices would have been the consideration of the patient. Hence, parents of a neonate with serious birth anomalies may not say, "Let the baby die; he will be a burden to us." Rather, they must make a decision in accord with the good of the child, weighing especially the fact that, in most cases, we judge life to be a gift worth preserving even if living may involve working with handicaps or infirmities. Because some parents abuse their rights to decide for their children, there is a trend to question the rights of parents to make proxy judgments and to insist on a better system of checks and balances than presently exists.

Discussion

Because of the nature of a proxy judgment, the person given the right to make such a judgment for another should be one who knows the person well and who has a loving concern for his or her well-being. Usually, then, the person who is presumed to have a legal and ethical right to make a proxy judgment is the parent, spouse, or next of kin; physicians and ethical or spiritual counselors should also be consulted, however.

The presumption that a parent, spouse, or relative will judge rightly is especially strong because of the bond of love that unites such a person to the patient. Of course, this presumption is not absolute. It may yield to a contrary fact. Thus, if the person who has the right to make this decision decides on something that does not seem to be in accord with the good of the patient, other responsible people may challenge the decision of the proxy and bring the matter before an ethics committee and, in some cases, before civil authorities. Physicians, nurses, and hospital administrators who determine with good reason that the proxy is not acting in accord with the patient's best interests have the ethical—and sometimes legal—obligation to intervene. If the case cannot be settled within the family and hospital community, the authority of the courts is often invoked.

The legal decisions mentioned in the introduction are examples of cases in which the courts intervened in the treatment of patients. Unfortunately, in the Saikewicz, Spring, and Fox decisions, the courts determined that only the legal authority can act as proxy for removing life-sustaining equipment in life or death situations. These decisions arrogate to public authority matters that belong in the private and personal domain and show a general lack of trust for loved ones to interpret the wishes of a comatose and, in these cases, dying person.

Conclusion

The aforementioned legal decisions were reached because the courts based their thinking on the notion that preserving life is an absolute good; thus, as the court stated in the Eichner case, the courts "have no choice but to intervene and examine each case on an individual patient-by-patient basis." Although preserving life is a highly valued good and when doubt exists the proxy should decide in favor of prolonging life, in some circumstances the proxy may determine ethically to allow a person to die because the therapy is ineffective or imposes a serious burden. For example, when prolonging life would not serve any human purpose or would impose an intolerable burden on the patient, the decision to withhold or remove life-supporting therapy may be made as long as the normal care due a sick person is maintained. Thus, a more nuanced ethical evaluation would have kept all of these cases out of court in the first place. Be that as it may, the usurpation by the courts of ethical decision making can be viewed only with great alarm.

Chapter 14 _____

Informed Consent and the Purpose of Medicine

The principle of informed consent is accepted widely as the norm that should guide decision making in the context of the patient-physician relationship. In brief, the principle requires the following: The physician must give sufficient information about proposed medical interventions to the person deciding about the use of the proposed interventions. The physician must help the person understand the information so that the decision made will be consistent with the person's own beliefs, goals, and values. The physician must ensure that the decision to consent to or refuse the proposed intervention is a free and voluntary choice by the person.

From an ethical perspective, observance of the principle of informed consent helps to foster the appropriate goals of the caregiving relationship in two ways. First, the principle focuses attention on the respect that is due to persons with regard to their right to choose their own goals and to make decisions to achieve those goals. Second, defining the roles and responsibilities of the persons in the caregiving relationship highlights the importance of a collaborative approach in making decisions about health care. Insofar as it functions in this manner, observing the principle of informed consent is crucial to striving for the appropriate goals of medicine. Misunderstanding of the principle, however, threatens to undermine the legitimate purposes of medicine and compromise the ethical integrity of individual practitioners as well.

Principles

Ethical or right action is action that seeks to respond to human needs in a way that promotes the "good" or fulfillment of the person. Within the specific context of health care, doing what is "good" for the person means doing that which contributes to the integrated functioning of the person so that the person is able to pursue life's goods and goals. This concept is also referred to as fulfilling the mission of life. When making decisions about the use or non-use of medical therapies, the primary question to be answered is, Will use of this therapy enable me to pursue the goods and goals of life—

my mission in life—to some degree? Consider, for example, the use of hemodialysis for a person suffering from renal failure. The fact that the procedure can keep the person alive may not sufficiently justify its use insofar as the person is concerned. Rather, the ability of the person to participate in life in a way that is fulfilling for the person is the norm for measuring the acceptability of chronic hemodialysis. Within this context, the ethical principle of informed consent identifies the conditions necessary for making decisions that contribute to the person's good, which help the person pursue the mission of life.

Discussion

In what appears to be an extension of the pervasive societal fascination with individual freedom and liberty, many people seek to define informed consent exclusively in terms of personal autonomy. As a result, many physicians think that regard for the principle of informed consent requires nothing more than a simple solicitation of and compliance with what the individual patient (or surrogate) wants or desires. This interpretation reflects the widely held societal belief that the "self" is all-important and is defined solely by its ability to choose its own values. Because personal preferences, which are highly idiosyncratic, are held to delimit the self, many people conclude that each self constitutes its own moral universe. Thus, self-fulfillment, according to this opinion, is a highly individualistic endeavor.

Two conclusions follow from this opinion. First, there is no objective basis for determining what is good or fulfilling with regard to persons. Hence, there are no objective criteria that can serve to guide or provide limits to individual decision making and choice. Second, the person exists in isolation. Relationship with others is desirable only insofar as the relationship furthers personal wants or desires. Thus, there is no basis for concern about the needs or good of the community of persons when seeking to achieve one's own good. When the meaning and requirements of informed consent are interpreted in this individualistic way, the reality of consent as a shared process of decision making is nullified. The physician becomes the mere instrument of the autonomous patient (or of the patient's surrogate). Medical decisions, selected from an individualistic perspective, may indeed be harmful to the patient insofar as he or she is a being with social responsibilities.

Consider the case of the irreversibly comatose person maintained on life support because "this is what the person wanted." Or consider the case of Janet Adkins who, upon learning that she was in the early stages of Alzheimer's disease, requested the help of a physician in bringing about her own death. In complying with Mrs. Adkins request, the physician argued that his action was justified because the physician's role is limited to carrying out the autonomously expressed wants and desires of the patient. In neither example is there any recognition that the physician has a responsibility to contribute to an understanding of what is good from the more objective social perspective and to help in determining appropriate means to promote the good. In other words, in both examples, the physician's role is limited to that of a technician.

In seeking to understand what the principle of informed consent requires of the physician, consideration of the patient's personal autonomy is important. The patient's autonomy is neither the primary nor the sole consideration, however. Correct understanding of informed consent requires and depends on an appreciation of something more. First, the good that is sought for an individual person is not only a personal good; we receive our concept of the good from society as well. What is good for the person is that which responds to human needs. These needs, however, are given with the nature of the human and are shared by all persons. Hence, it is within the community of persons that we come to understand what is good, what contributes to human fulfillment. Accordingly, our society seeks to prevent suicide because we know that suicide is not an appropriate response to human need. It is not an act that promotes the social good of the person. Suicide is harmful to the individual person and to the community of persons as well. Second, an assessment of the ability of a proposed medical therapy to enable an individual person to pursue the mission of life must take place in a societal context. This contextual assessment is required because the person pursues life's mission as a member of community. Thus, the understanding of informed consent as a shared process of decision making is quite appropriate. The role of the physician is correctly interpreted in light of this understanding.

Conclusion

In the caregiving relationship and in the decision-making process, the physician does provide technical expertise and must be competent in doing so. The physician enters the relationship not just as technician, however, but as a fellow member of the community of persons. Thus, the physician is responsible to help the patient discern what is good in light of the community's understanding of the good. In addition, the physician must help the person assess actions taken to promote that good not only insofar as those actions affect the individual person but also as they affect the community.

Chapter 15 _____

Standards for Surrogates

With increasing frequency, family members and other surrogates are faced with choices about treatment options for patients who, because of incapacity, cannot choose on their own behalf. Such was the case when Bonnie Keiner requested the removal of life support from her mother, Dorothy Longway. Mrs. Longway was irreversibly comatose as a result of extensive neurologic damage following a series of strokes. Her daughter petitioned the courts to allow her to make this treatment decision for her mother. In offering its opinion in the case, the Illinois Supreme Court raised the following questions: According to what standard(s) should such surrogate decisions be made? How can Dorothy Longway's interests be furthered appropriately when she herself cannot participate in the decision-making process?

Principles

The standards that generally guide decision making for the incompetent person in the health care context have a long legal history. The principles of "substitute judgment" and "best interests" were developed originally to instruct guardians in handling financial and property decisions for the incompetent.[1] Today, these same principles are applied when choices about medical care and therapy must be made for patients who lack decisional capacity. Although both standards are designed to support the basic values underlying informed consent in general (i.e., the welfare of the patient and patient self-determination), there are significant differences owing to the fact of incapacity.

Using the substitute judgment standard as a guide, surrogate decision makers are instructed to choose as the patient would choose if he or she were able. Thus, decisions about treatment options under this standard should further the well-being of the patient in light of the patient's own understanding of what constitutes well-being. What this approach requires, of course, is knowledge of the patient's preferences, values, commitments, and concerns. Explicit written statements by the patient him or herself (e.g., a living will) may seem to be the most reliable source of information regarding treatment preferences. However, lifestyle, past choices and behaviors, and the kinds and qualities of relationships the person developed can also provide reliable insights into the patient's preferences.

When no evidence exists about the patient's desires, the principle that guides surrogate decision making is the patient's "best interest." Adopting the perspective of a "reasonable person," the surrogate is directed to choose options that would most likely contribute to the patient's well-being. This principle aims at objectivity by relying on considerations of "relief of suffering, the preservation or restoration of functioning, and the quality as well as the extent of life sustained"[2] to define the limits of "well-being."

Although these principles become operative at different times according to the circumstances of the patient, both are oriented toward promoting the good and well-being of the patient in question.

Discussion

In allowing for the removal of the life-sustaining therapy in the Longway case, the Supreme Court of Illinois accepted the substitute judgment offered by Mrs. Longway's daughter on Mrs. Longway's behalf. Unlike other courts (e.g., the New York Court of Appeals), the Illinois high court did not require prior explicit written documentation to allow a substitute judgment decision. The court recognized that Mrs. Longway's life goals, values, and preferences could be the controlling factors in the present treatment decision even though Mrs. Longway was unable to participate actively in the process because the decisions were being made by her daughter who loved her and had a lifetime of experience observing her mother fashion her own life according to those values and goals.

Some courts, however, in attempting to guard against error and the possible intrusion of subjectivity into the surrogate's decision, have not allowed the substitute judgment principle to serve as the standard. Thus, even in cases in which family members were willing and able to make substitute judgment decisions, some were not allowed to do so because the courts did not find that lifestyle, past conversations about sickness and death, past health care practices, and so forth provided clear and convincing evidence of the patient's preferences and values.[3] Because the patient, while competent, did not write down specific directions about the use or non-use of life-sustaining treatments, the best interests standard was held to be the appropriate guide for decision making.

In something of an aberration, the Missouri Supreme Court in the case of Nancy Beth Cruzan dismissed both standards for surrogate decision making and argued that incompetent persons who have not left prior written directives about medical care surrender the right to have decisions made in accord with their own values and preferences. In these circumstances, the court contended, the state should intervene and determine treatment in light of the state's interests and values. This opinion undermines the consent process by denying that the values of the patient in question ought to set the parameters within which treatment decisions are made.

What of the other approaches, however? Clearly, when little or nothing is known about the patient, the best interests standard is the appropriate guide for decision making. In such cases, every effort should be made to ensure that the patient's best interests and well-being are the controlling concerns rather than the surrogate's biases or the health care practitioner's view of what is "best."

When the lifestyle, attitudes, views, and values of the patient in question are known by others, especially by family members, substitute judgment should be the standard applied in treatment decisions. Written documentation by the patient, although helpful, ought not to be required before this standard is invoked.

Conclusion

The goal of all decision making in medicine and health care is to make choices that support and are consistent with the values and preferences of the patient. The fact of incapacity should not negate a lifetime of prior choice. Relying on the substitute judgment standard whenever possible can help to ensure that the patient's personal value system is the controlling concern in important treatment decisions.

Notes

1. President's Commission for the Study of Ethical Problems in Medicine and Biomedical and Behavioral Research, *Making Health Care Decisions* (Washington, D.C.: U.S. Government Printing Office, 1982), 177.
2. Ibid., 180.
3. In re O'Connor, 72 N.Y. 2d 517, N.E. 2d Dist., 534 N.Y.S. 2d 886 (1988).

Chapter 16 _____

Informed Consent: Therapeutic and Nontherapeutic Procedures

The federal agency that protects human research subjects from harm recently criticized a clinical research study at the University of California at Los Angeles.[1] In that study, medication was withdrawn from persons being treated for schizophrenia to determine whether they would do better without the medication. Several of the patients had more than one severe relapse, including hallucinations and paranoia; one participant even committed suicide. All of the participants signed informed consent documents. Some critics of the research program—especially family members of patients in the program—thought the research should never have been approved. This case presents an opportunity to examine the ethical norms of informed consent, especially the ethical norms for informed consent in clinical trials.

Principles

The ethical mandate of informed consent arises from the goals of the physician-patient relationship. The remote goal of this relationship is the overall well-being of the patient. The proximate goal is the health of the patient. Thus, as Leon Kass, a physician-philosopher at the University of Chicago, maintains, the physician is concerned with "the well-working of the enlivened body and its power to sense, think, feel, desire, move, and maintain self." As result of an examination of the enlivened body, the physician offers the patient a medical diagnosis as the first step in striving for the proximate goal of their relationship, the health of the patient.

To further the quest for the proximate goal of the physician-patient relationship, however, the physician also offers a plan of medical or surgical therapy designed to preserve or restore health. The diagnosis and prognosis must be presented to the patient in language the patient can understand. The remote goal of the relationship—the patient's overall well-being—must also be considered, however. A person who understands the diagnosis and prognosis may determine that the medical plan is too expensive or would interfere with other important goods and goals that contribute to his or her overall well-being. For this reason, the patient renders the final decision with regard to the use of medical or surgical procedures. That is, the patient, either implicitly or explicitly, compares the particular goods associated with striving for health with the other goods for which the patient habitually strives.

Suppose for example, a woman has been striving for years to save money to educate her grandchildren. Informed that she would have to devote all her savings to a medical plan to overcome a recently diagnosed cancer, she decides to forego medical treatment and "let nature take its course," thus assuring the good of a college education for her grandchildren.

As we posit that the ultimate responsibility for decision making rests with the patient, let us also emphasize that the role of the physician involves more than simply presenting options to the patient. The physician is dedicated to the *good* of the patient. Thus, the options presented to the patient should be presented in light of the patient's health and overall well-being.

Another way to envision the informed consent process is to realize that each person has biological, emotional, social, and creative (spiritual) functions. Physicians are experts with regard to the biological and emotional functions. Patients, however, are experts in regard to their social and creative functions—which are the integrating and value-centered functions of human well-being. Although physicians will have some general notions about the social and creative goods that integrate most persons' quests for well-being, they will not possess accurate knowledge about a particular person's values and goods insofar as social and creative needs are concerned. Thus, the patient has freedom to accept or reject the physician's recommendations in accord with his or her habitually determined goods and goals.

In contemporary America, the purpose and process of informed consent is often described as an effort to "assure patient autonomy." Actually, this description is a limited and misleading concept of informed consent. If we envision the informed consent process as a collaborative process with a twofold purpose, the process is concerned with more than autonomy on the part of the patient.

Does the ethical responsibility to work for the good of particular patients pertain as well to physicians engaged in clinical research? Physician-researchers are physician first and foremost; they are researchers only secondarily. Physicians-researchers should not envision their research subjects as a large group who may be subjected to harm so that the researcher can obtain general information. One expert in legal and medical ethics sums up the responsibility of the physician in clinical research trials by stating, "The subject should be no worse off in a clinical trial than if using accepted therapy."[2]

Discussion

Does the foregoing analysis imply that a subject in a research program may never be allowed to accept a risk of harm or injury? To answer this question, we must invoke a classic distinction between therapeutic and nontherapeutic research. Therapeutic research, or clinical research, aims at the health and well-being of particular patients. It is a combination of therapy and research. The goal of therapy—benefit for an individual patient—must always take precedence in clinical research. Risk of harm or injury is an intrinsic factor in any therapeutic intervention. Often the risk of harm or injury is so minimal it is not considered by the researcher or patient. At other times, the risk of harm may be more serious. The patient may accept or reject the more serious risk by comparing it with other goods of life. Even if risks are included in the protocol, however, the protocol for clinical research should never involve a therapy that of itself offers less than standard treatment. Even if a double blind protocol is employed, the patients in the control group (the group that does not receive the drug or therapy being evaluated) should receive a drug or therapy that meets the norms for standard treatment.

Nontherapeutic research has an entirely different purpose. Whereas therapeutic research or clinical research aims at preserving or restoring the health of individual participants in the research program, nontherapeutic research aims at obtaining knowledge that will be utilized for the health of people in the future. Although nontherapeutic research is an important humanistic endeavor, it aims at the well-being of the community, not the health or well-being of the individual. The ethical norms for nontherapeutic research do allow a subject to accept a risk of harm. In these cases, however, the subject should be informed clearly that the research protocol is nontherapeutic.

Subjecting oneself to a risk of serious harm in a nontherapeutic research project is an act of altruism and self-giving. Although a proxy may give consent to benefit a ward, the proxy does not have the right to place a ward at risk on the grounds of altruism or self abnegation. For this reason, the selection of subjects for nontherapeutic research should be a very stringent process. Subjects in nontherapeutic research projects that involve risk of serious harm or injury should not be minors or persons who are impaired insofar as making competent judgments are concerned. Researchers tend to confuse the two types of research and apply the ethical norms for nontherapeutic research to therapeutic research—as the Tuskeegee study, which deprived black men suffering from syphilis of penicillin that would have cured their disease, and the UCLA of Alzheimer's disease indicate.

Conclusion

The researchers studying the effect of withdrawing medicine from persons suffering from schizophrenia did not design a protocol to help the individuals enrolled in the program. Any benefit from this research project would mainly be for people in the future. UCLA's institutional review board—the internal study group that evaluates all research projects—should not have approved this project. Not only did the project allow patients to be worse off than they would have been under standard therapy, it also subjected people who were doubtfully capable of offering informed consent to serious harm in nontherapeutic research.

Notes

1. Philip Hilts, "Agency Faults a UCLA Study for Suffering of Mental Patients," *New York Times,* March 9, 1994.
2. Jay Katz, "Human Experimentation and Human Rights," *St. Louis Law Review* (fall 1993): 30.

Chapter 17 _____

Informed Consent: Neonatal Care

Sheila Clifford weighed 1,000 grams when she was born prematurely. Because of her precarious hold on life, she was flown ninety miles to a hospital with a neonatal intensive care unit (NICU), where more thorough and advanced medical therapy was available. Anyone observing the clinical activity upon Sheila's arrival at the NICU would have been impressed with the medical team's care and concern for her. Equally impressive was the care offered by pastoral care personnel and social workers when her parents arrived at the hospital. A sincere effort was made to consider their spiritual and temporal concerns arising from Sheila's condition. Not much time was spent conferring with the parents about medical management plans, however. Life-saving procedures were explained, but permission to initiate and continue these procedures was seldom requested.

If the definitions of informed consent formulated by some contemporary ethicists were accepted as the norm, the conclusion could be drawn that in neonatal care units, the rights of parents are sometimes violated. According to these ethicists, health care professionals are responsible only to carry out the "autonomous" directives of patients or their proxies. If there would be any disagreement, the directives of the parents should prevail. This chapter considers the issue of caring for infants in the NICU, seeking to explain why the medical team on occasion assumes more responsibility for decision making than do medical teams caring for patients in other settings.

Principles

To understand the ethical responsibilities of any profession, one must have a clear understanding of the objectives of the profession. Only then may one proceed to state the ethical norms for the profession. By fulfilling the ethical norms of a profession, one not only serves the client or patient in need of help from the professional, one also fulfills oneself as a person and develops the skills and virtues proper to the profession.

What are the objectives of the medical personnel on a neonatal care team? Certainly, they provide health care for infants and children at the request of the parents. They also care for infants as agents of the community or society. Society needs healthy children. Society strives to foster the well-being of children, especially the weaker ones. When infants are born in a debilitated condition, not only their parents but society at large has an interest in ensuring that the ailing infants will become as strong and healthy as possible. In a very real sense, neonatologists and pediatricians are the delegates of society. They have a direct responsibility to the child that does not stem entirely from the parents. The philosophy behind this delegation and the desire for children to be strong and healthy is not based on a perverted notion that the child exists for the society. Rather, the delegation results from the assumption that society exists for the individual. Hence, society should support facilities and professions that promote the well-being of individuals—especially the well-being of children.

Maintaining that medical personnel caring for infants and children receive a mandate from society as well as from the parents does not pre-empt the responsibilities of parents. Parents are also advocates for their children. This mandate does indicate, however, that decision making concerning medical therapy for infants and children is a collaborative process. The unifying theme of this collaboration is that parents and medical personnel have an ethical responsibility to strive for the overall well-being of the infant or child.

Discussion

Given that medical personnel as well as parents are advocates for children, what implications follow?

Medical personnel and parents alike should be concerned with the overall well-being of the child—not only with the possibility of keeping the child alive. Overall well-being is very difficult to judge, especially for infants, but it involves more than mere physiological function. In addition to the function of the infant, medical personnel consider social and economic factors as they assess well-being. In some cases, especially if severe neurological deprivation is evident, continuing life support clearly does not provide overall benefit for the infant. Yet, simply because an infant is physically or mentally impaired does not justify withholding life support. Traditional ethical norms for withholding or withdrawing life support should be utilized: Does this therapy impose a severe burden on the patient? Will this therapy be effective or ineffective insofar as the overall well-being of the patient is concerned?

Applying these ethical norms to infants is much more difficult than applying them to other persons. The prognosis for infants is always tinged with uncertainty. Every neonatal care professional can cite a case in which an infant survived and thrived contrary to professional expectations. Moreover, when judging the future well-being of a disabled infant, we must not underestimate the value of human life. Adults with genetic or acquired anomalies are vociferous in appealing for life support for debilitated infants. In making difficult ethical decisions, medical personnel caring for infants and children often have a greater responsibility toward their patients than do medical personnel caring for older patients.

States and cities should give high priority to the health and well-being of their children. Realizing that society has a special interest in the health of children logically leads to the question: Is enough attention and funding devoted by society to the health needs of children? Based on every survey and study available, the answer is no. Although society fulfills its responsibility to some extent with regard to acute care, primary preventative services, follow-up rehabilitation, and chronic care services are lacking.

In our pragmatic society the notion of protecting and enhancing the life of weak and debilitated infants might become unpopular. In the near future prolonging the life of impaired infants will be considered by some people to be wasteful and ridiculous. Because of the ability to detect genetic anomalies and other pathologies before birth, there is a growing tendency to recommend the abortion of less-than-perfect infants. Ethically responsible health care professionals march to the beat of a different drummer, however. As Karl Barth, the noted Protestant theologian, stated:

> No society whether family, village or state, is really strong if it will not carry its weak and even its weakest members. They belong to it no less than the strong, and the quiet work of their maintenance and care which might seem useless on a superficial level, is perhaps more effective than labor, culture, or productivity in knitting it closely and securely together. On the other hand, a community which regards and treats its weak members as a hindrance or even proceeds to their extermination is on the verge of collapse.[1]

Conclusion

Sheila Clifford survived and is thriving today. Far from signifying a violation of parents rights to informed consent, the prompt and aggressive medical care given to Sheila indicated a collaborative approach to her overall well-being. This approach is based on the love parents have for their children but also on the responsibility of health care professionals to foster the future well-being of society.

Note

1. Karl Barth, *Church Dogmatics,* Vol. III, no. 4, (Grand Rapids, MI: Eerdmans, 1978): 424.

Chapter 18 _____

When Children Can Consent

On August 21, 1994, sixteen-year-old Benito Agrelo peacefully and silently died in his mother's loving embrace. Benito's death marked the end of a life dominated by surgeries, transplants, and medications for a diseased liver. Yet the events leading up to Benito's passage into that good night were far from gentle. Only two months prior to his death, the Florida Department of Health and Rehabilitative Services forcibly removed Benito, kicking and screaming, from his home after learning that he had discontinued the immunosuppressant drugs used to prevent rejection of his second transplanted liver. The state sought to resume drug therapy to prolong the boy's life. A judge in the case decided that Benito had a right to forego the medicine, which caused severe headaches, nausea, irritability, and a host of other side effects. Did Benito in fact have a moral right to stop treatment knowing that death would ensue? What role does the adolescent play in such a decision vis-a-vis his parents and the state? Did Benito have a special responsibility to endure the side effects given the fact that this was the second liver transplant he had received?

Principles

In the past few decades, society and the law have increasingly recognized the rights and responsibilities of minors in medical decision making. The trend to incorporate minors in treatment decisions demonstrates a positive respect for the intrinsic freedom and dignity of the child, as well as a recognition of an emerging developmental capability to make important decisions. No longer can children be seen but not heard. In most cases parents give permission for treatment for their minor children—but children are also now asked to assent or agree to the treatment proposal. In some cases the law has recognized a variety of circumstances wherein the autonomy of minors allows them to give actual consent to medical decisions, rather than just assent. Emancipated minors (those who are married, are parents, or are living apart from the family in a financially secure way) can legally give consent to treatment. In most states, legal minor treatment statutes allow minors to consent to certain treatments without parental permission (e.g., abortions, contraceptives, and treatments for sexually transmitted diseases and drug addiction). Finally, mature minor statutes allow adolescents to consent to treatments if they have demonstrated sufficient maturity to fulfill the requirements of giving informed consent.

Nevertheless this ever-increasing embodiment of legal recognition does not necessarily guarantee that ethical consent is being actualized when minors are allowed to make decisions for themselves. The law may provide some boundaries for decision making, but health care professionals must prudently apply the laws. For example, the law recognizes adult status at the age of 18. Yet, a particular minor who is 17 years, 360 days old may possess a much better ability to make informed consent than someone who has just turned 20. Moreover, although one might not be able to give aspirin to a 12 year old without parental permission, it may be possible to give her contraceptives. Thus, the law offers some glaring inconsistencies when juxtaposed with traditional criteria for ethical informed consent (with the exception, perhaps, of mature minor statutes in which actual competency is assessed). Therefore, the health care team should evaluate minors on a case-by-case basis to ascertain whether they can give ethical consent.

What capabilities associated with consent should the health care professional look for in the minor? Informed consent has traditionally included the three components of information, understanding, and freedom. The minor needs to have knowledge of his or her diagnosis and prognosis, the nature of the proposed tests or treatments, the risks and benefits of such procedures, and potential alternatives. The minor must be able to understand what this knowledge means and be able to reason about possible alternatives in light of his or her goals or purpose in life. Minors often lack this capacity because they can focus only on immediate consequences of pain and suffering rather than integrating any temporary discomfort into an overall view of life. Perhaps a standard to employ would be whether one would feel comfortable with an adult who would make the same decision for the same reasons. Finally, the minor must be free from coercive forces that might impinge on his or her autonomy. Is the minor sufficiently independent of parental and physician hegemony to consent without feeling he or she has to do something out of fear of alienating parents or the doctor? Such a concern might arise in the case of a fifteen-year-old Jehovah's Witness refusing a blood transfusion. Has the minor freely ratified the decision to be a Jehovah's Witness and follow the religion's tenets, or is the decision tied more to parental belief and fear of alienation from his or her worshiping community? A fifteen-year-old *can* embrace the tenets of his or her faith, but one must proceed with caution in evaluating the capacity to consent.

Is there a threshold, minimum age for informed consent? Developmental psychology suggests that around the age of thirteen to fourteen, minors may develop the capacity to make informed consent. The minor's ability to navigate the transition from assent to consent will depend on his or her maturity and life experience. The minor's capability to give consent is also predicated on the severity of the disease and the complexity of treatment required. A young minor may be able to consent to taking tetracycline for a flare-up of acne but less able to consent to using isotretinoin (accutane) for cystic acne (which entails more deleterious side effects). A minor may be able to consent to the surgical removal of a mole, but a decision regarding the discontinuation of chemotherapy for a deadly cancer may stretch the child's ability to make a free and informed decision. Moreover, such decisions ideally will be made in consultation with the parents—if only because they may be the party responsible for payment for the treatments.

Another caveat deserves mention. In the zeal to promote the principle of autonomy in minors, is the minor child inappropriately saddled with decisions that would tax the decision-making capabilities of most adults? One should not precipitously ascribe decision-making capability to children, lest we place an undue burden on them.

When a minor lacks the ability to give informed consent and parental permission is needed, health care professionals nevertheless should integrate the minor into the decision-making process by means of minor assent. This process involves helping the child to know and understand his or her condition and the proposed treatment and what he or she will likely experience. One should also attempt to elicit the child's permission to proceed with treatment when possible. In doing so, one provides the foundations from which the minor can grow gradually into a legitimately autonomous decision maker.

Discussion

Given this background, how should we evaluate the decision of Benito Agrelo and the other parties involved? Benito's longstanding battle with his liver disease and the side effects of the medication indicate that his experience gave him an improved ability to know what the prescribed treatment involved. Benito had seen many of his friends who had received transplants die, so he was not unacquainted with the reality of death. Benito himself stated, "I should have the right to make my own decision. I know the consequences; I know the problems." The judge in the case interviewed Benito for an extended period of time and listened to several hours of testimony from the treating physicians before arriving at his conclusion that Benito in fact possessed the capacity to give informed consent in discontinuing his anti-rejection medication. Moreover, Benito exhibited a freedom to consent without coercion from parents or physicians. On the surface, Benito seemed best able to judge the nature of his quality of life and the possibility of success of the treatment. He seemed best able to judge the burdens associated with the treatment in comparison with the benefits it offered. Was the decision not reasonable? Many adults in similar situations refuse treatment because of untoward side effects of a similar magnitude and debilitating effect. Although the state has an interest in intervening in decisions when the minor's best interests are not being actualized, that scenario did not seem to be the case in the Agrelo situation.

Despite this analysis, some questions remain. For example, Benito's decision to curtail medication and then discontinue it completely in October of 1993 without physician consultation calls into question the maturity of the parties involved. Were there other alternatives? Could a different immunosuppressant drug have been utilized? Moreover, in accepting a second liver, did Benito implicitly accept a greater responsibility to endure side effects? There is much debate about the ethics of retransplantation when a patient such as Benito receives a second organ while others die on the waiting list in anticipation of their first transplant. Regardless of the ethics of retransplantation, did Benito not have a greater obligation to preserve a scarce resource once he made a decision to accept it? Would it have been appropriate to place him back on drug therapy, with an increased effort to treat the side effects and reevaluate six months later? If the side effects were still too burdensome, the medication could have been stopped at that point.

Conclusion

Health care professionals and the law increasingly are recognizing minors' ability and even right to make medical decisions for themselves. This movement seems ethically acceptable when the requirements of informed consent are fulfilled. However, the complexity of adolescent decisional capacity, requires careful scrutiny on a case-by-case basis dependent on the maturity of the child and the seriousness of the illness. These types of decisions require prudence to avoid the errors of treating emerging adults as children or prematurely granting the status of adulthood to children.

Chapter 19 _____

Telling the Truth to Patients

"What to tell the patient" has been considered one of the more difficult and delicate ethical questions for health care professionals. In the not-too-distant past, some physicians and other health care professionals thought that the less patients knew about their condition, the better would be their chances of recovery. Some health care professionals would even withhold information about impending death, fearing that such knowledge might lead a person to despair. Because of an awakened moral sense on the part of health care professionals and a sharper realization that patients have legal and moral rights that must be respected, there is now a much greater tendency to be open and honest concerning patients' conditions, the purpose of the proposed treatment, and the treatment prognosis. The Patient's Bill of Rights of the American Hospital Association states:

> The patient has the right to obtain from the physician complete current information concerning diagnosis, treatment, and prognosis in terms the patient can be reasonably expected to understand.

Principles

Clearly, information on serious sickness or impending death must be furnished even if the individual does not ask for it. Legal precedent as well as moral concern prompts this realization. Hence, physicians and other health care professionals may not defend their lack of communication by pleading that the patient did not wish to know and did not ask questions. In some hospitals, a patients' representative helps patients understand their situation, especially when surgery is anticipated. Whenever possible, the leader of the health care team—the physician—should be involved in explaining the situation to the patient.

Although health care professionals usually respect patients' rights insofar as providing the proper information, difficult situations often arise in which health care professionals hesitate to tell patients their true condition.

For example, patients with serious cases of cancer might become despondent and even suicidal if they knew their true situation. With this in mind, The Patient's Bill of Rights states:

> When it is not medically advisable to give such information to the patient, the information should be made available to an appropriate person in his or her behalf.

Discussion

Although well-intentioned, the foregoing statement is unsatisfactory and incomplete. It seems to indicate that when health care professionals feel that harm might result if the patient knows the truth, they fulfill their obligation by telling a friend or family member about the patient's condition and prognosis. The statement does not indicate, however, what the family member or the friend is supposed to do once the information has been communicated. To ensure proper respect for the patient, another dimension of the situation must be explored.

Even though the medical personnel might fear untoward results if patients are informed of their true condition, they should not conclude that patients should never be told the truth. Indeed, in these cases health care professionals should remember the words of Eric Cassell:

> The depression in patients that commonly occurs after the diagnosis of a fatal disease seems to stem in part from the conspiracy of silence. The physician can be a great help by simply making it clear to the patient that he is available for open and direct communication.[1]

Interviews with ill or dying patients reveal that they do not wish to be kept continually in doubt about their condition; on the other hand, they do not want it revealed to them in an abrupt or brutal manner. According to Howard Brody:

> A decision to reveal a grave prognosis, which may be "ethical" in itself, may become "unethical" if the physician tells the patient bluntly and then withdraws, without offering any emotional support to help the patient resolve his feelings. In fact, the assurance that the physician plans to see it through along with the patient, and that he will always make himself available to offer any comfort possible, may be more important than the bad news itself. In many of the "sour cases" that are offered as justification for withholding the truth, it may well be the absence of this transmission of com-

passion, rather than the telling of the truth, that produced the unfortunate result.[2]

Because physicians are not always able to convey information concerning serious illness or impending death in a fitting manner, a person trained in the dynamics of accepting sickness and death is useful in the present-day hospital setting. Crisis counseling of this nature is not an arcane art, but one must be prepared competently in order to perform it well. Well-meaning but untrained people can do more harm than good when trying to help in crises.

Conclusion

Because of the general public's increased knowledge of psychology and greater regard for the subjective process that accompanies sickness and dying, the ethical question in regard to truth telling has changed. The question should not be, "Should we tell?" but "How do we share this information with the patient?"

Notes

1. Eric Cassell, *The Healer's Art* (Philadelphia: J.B. Lippincott, 1976), 197.
2. Howard Brody, *Ethical Decisions in Medicine* (Boston: Little, Brown & Co., 1976), 40.

Chapter 20

Confidentiality

From the Hippocratic oath to modern ethical codes, confidentiality has been a concern in health care. The fundamental aim of confidentiality is to protect patients from the revelation of important, sometimes intimate, information that if made public, would damage the person's reputation.

Confidentiality is a concern for lawyers, teachers, and other professionals; because the medical relationship is especially sensitive, however, confidentiality with regard to patients' diagnoses and prognoses is especially important. Thus, in an effort to foster trust, confidentiality excludes unauthorized persons from gaining access to patient information and requires that people who have such information legitimately refrain from communicating it to others.

Numerous examples of the difficulty of protecting confidential information have surfaced. Recently a technician leaked information about a possible bone marrow donor in California to a young man dying of leukemia in Texas. Court battles were waged for two months because of this breach of confidential records stored in a university computer bank. Does a minor have the right to physician consultation and confidentiality without parental involvement when birth control devices are desired? What are the rights of psychiatric patients with regard to access to their files? Can third-party payers demand a copy of the patient's medical records before payment is made? In modern technological medicine, how many people actually have access to a patient's records? One survey estimated that at least seventy-five people need access to provide quality care.

Are the foregoing questions indications that confidentiality can no longer be guaranteed and is therefore a defunct ethical requirement in the medical profession?

Principles

Confidentiality in the medical transaction can be crucial to the goals of the physician and the patient. If the patient does not believe that the physician will maintain confidences, he or she may not supply possibly embarrassing or personal information that is important for good history-taking and diagnostic procedures. Likewise, confidentiality is important during the treatment period because physician-patient interactions depend on trust. This crucial element of trust in the physician-patient relationship could be damaged in the overall concern for a patient's health. Several relationships are at stake if trust is broken: the patient-physician relationship, the patient's relationships with other health care providers, the reputation of the physician in the community, and the physician's relationship with other patients. Ultimately, privacy, personal autonomy, the decision-making process for physician and patient, the patient's responsibility for his or her own health, and public health values could be threatened.

Discussion

Often many people need access to medical records to ensure proper care for patients. In health care facilities where teams of healers provide care, all team members must have access to needed information. Groups of subspecialists, attending physicians, medical students, three shifts of nurses, and a variety of auxiliary services—each necessary to care for a patient— must have access to records that chart the patient's progress. Simplistic solutions to the issue of confidentiality should be avoided. It would be dangerous to isolate information into different compartments, as if the patient were not a whole person or as if one could cure the person by attending only to the physical, social, or psychological dimensions of the patient's life. Although many providers may be involved in care, neither idle curiosity nor simple interest is sufficient reason to have access to a patient's chart. Administrative auditors who have some need to examine a chart and health care professionals on the floor who are caring for the patient must keep this principle in mind. Better health care through multiple specialists, especially in a university setting, must balance carefully the patient's right to confidentiality and the need for information.

Computerization of medical records also increases the potential for breaches of confidentiality. Although the latest technology may make storage and retrieval of valuable information more efficient and less cumbersome, the director of medical records must provide a network to protect privacy. Physicians may usually depend on this network when they are in an institutional setting, but they should remember that in private practice it is their responsibility to ensure the safety of this information. This protection of records may be difficult when a central computer bank is used— especially when not all the users are physicians.

Another issue that is more controllable is the self-discipline required by all health care workers when dealing with patient information. Where something is said—in the cafeteria, in the hall, in the elevator—can be crucial. It is not ethical to allow indiscriminate conversation that violates any patient's right to confidentiality to take place in or out of health care facilities. This reminder is pertinent with cases used in classrooms, rounds, literature, and other teaching areas. One should be careful to mask the identity of patients whose cases are used to respect their right to confidentiality.

Confidentiality has its limits. Increased access is the result of modern medicine because quality care is ensured only if a larger number of people have access to a patient's chart. Without greater access, care could be compromised. Classic cases limit the responsibility of confidentiality: When a patient threatens suicide, for example, confidentiality must be broken to prevent harm to the patient and to other members of society. Such a threat may even be an indirect plea for help. Similarly, public health laws require a breaking of confidentiality to prevent harm to society or to innocent third parties. Such is the case with suspected child abuse, contagious disease, or persons that threaten the life of other members of society.

Conclusion

Confidentiality is meant to protect persons and the relationships that they have with health care providers, to ensure trust and patient autonomy, and to provide security as health care is provided. Modern technological medicine poses a new challenge to older concepts of confidentiality narrowly inscribed in the one-on-one model of health care. Nonetheless, the values that confidentiality was supposed to foster still exist, and their protection must be reexamined in contemporary settings so that the patient's health may continue to be served.

Chapter 21

Confidentiality in the Computer Age

Modern technology enables us to transmit information over phone lines, access computer files from distant locations, and store huge amounts of data on disks small enough to slip into our pockets. These capabilities—and the rapidly expanding information superhighway—have many benefits for patient care, but they also have patient advocates worried. In 1993 burglars stole computer disks containing the names of 8,000 patients from a Florida AIDS clinic. In another case, a banker cross-referenced a list of patients with cancer against a list of people who had outstanding loans at his bank and then called in the loans. In 1996, twenty-four people in Maryland were indicted in connection with a scheme in which clerks sold information about identified individual patients, obtained from the state's Medicaid data base, to four health maintenance organizations.

The Joint Commission on Accreditation of Healthcare Organizations requires facilities to have safeguards in place to protect the security of computerized and paper-based medical records. Yet more than a quarter of the people responding to a 1993 Harris poll said that information about them had been improperly disclosed. Legislation designed to protect medical-record privacy is pending before the U.S. Senate, but state laws vary widely with regard to the kinds of disclosure they allow and their requirements for patient consent. In spite of the computer's obvious value in the health care setting, its use is also replete with problems—the greatest being the threat to confidentiality.

Principles

One of the most important obligations of health care professionals to patients is the protection of confidences. The fundamental aim of confidentiality is to guard people from the unauthorized release of sensitive information that might be harmful to their reputation. Trust between health care professionals and patients is rooted in the promise that intimate information will be treated with respect and will be shared only with those who need to know.

Confidentiality has never been an absolute requirement, however, nor would that be desirable. Patients willingly permit the therapeutic use of information in the hope of improving the outcomes of their treatments. Some people even participate in research to help others with the same condition. In potentially dangerous situations, the family or society may have an obligation to breach confidentiality in order to prevent harm either to the patient or to the public.

Generally, health care professionals seek informed consent before releasing or sharing medical information. If the information is going to be stored in a computerized database, we either strip it of identifiers or ask patients for consent each time the data is used for new purposes. Electronic medical records present ethical challenges because tremendous amounts of sensitive information will be available to large numbers of people, and geographic distance will not be a factor. The threat to confidentiality will grow as genetic testing becomes more common. It will be increasingly important to consider the balance between the right of privacy and the potential benefit or harm to others. The stakes are high: Sensitive information in the wrong hands might have negative implications for employment and housing.

Discussion

Every time a person consults a health care professional, is admitted to a hospital, or undergoes a medical test, a written or computerized record is created or an entry is made to an existing record. Billions of such medical records exist in the United States, most of which will be retained for 10–25 years. Many of these records contain very personal information: documentation of treatment of alcoholism, past drug use, genetic predispositions to various diseases. Yet most records are available to many users for a variety of legitimate as well as questionable purposes. The American College of Healthcare Administrators estimates that seventy-five persons have access to any patient record. The Institute of Medicine (IOM) states that the number of parties with a need to know is so large that it would not even attempt to provide a complete list.

Large computerized information networks give providers and payers instant access to personal health data. In 1991 IOM released an influential report, *The Computer-Based Patient Record: An Essential Technology for Health Care*. It advocates the adoption of the computer-based patient record as standard medical practice in the United States. Such a record would be a continuous chronological history of a patient's medical care linked to various aids, such as reminders and alerts to clinicians.

Making medical information more accessible empowers patients. Computers help people acquire medical information, interact with caregivers, connect with support groups, and even carry out a treatment plan. When a patient's record is not stored in a computer, important information may be lost, unreadable, or unavailable at the moment it is most needed. The patient also loses the benefits of software programs that monitor drug interactions and provide on-line consultations.

In some situations, the computer can actually increase confidentiality by requiring the use of passwords and recording the names of persons who look at confidential information. In addition, the widespread collection of health information could result in a national health care database. Doctors in emergency rooms could access information about a patient from another part of the country; public health officials could track epidemics more effectively; and researchers could scan the population to identify risk factors that increase a person's chance of getting certain types of cancer.

Although such technology would probably mean better continuity and quality of care, it could also increase the difficulty of keeping sensitive medical information confidential. Passwords are notoriously easy to guess or steal, and so-called firewalls of protection have been breached by hackers who have no motivation other than to see what is on the other side. Others may have strong economic incentives for viewing confidential information. Pharmaceutical firms building direct-mail advertising for new drugs might be very interested in the names and addresses of people taking competing medications. Life insurance companies could save money if they knew in advance which of their applicants were likely to get sick or die.

Even before the introduction of the computer, serious inroads on confidentiality appeared. With the current restructuring of the health care delivery system, people obtain their health care in a variety of settings and from a growing number of professionals. Computers link geographically separate facilities and allow physicians to access remote data. As health care is increasingly provided through such integrated networks, traditional standards of confidentiality will be further diminished unless patients are given some form of control over access to their records. Computer-based patient records will not only be seen by more parties but also will contain a wider array of data. Parties who *desire* to know will vie with those who truly *need* to know. Advocates argue that unrestricted access facilitates the efficient provision of health care. That claim, however—even if true—must be weighed against the invasion of privacy, the damage to the physician-patient relationship, and the potential for abuse.

In an article about the privacy of personal information in a new health care system, Lawrence Gostin acknowledged the conflict between privacy and extensive data collection but found the benefits of such data collection worth the price in loss of privacy: "A health care system supported by data on almost any relevant subject, accessible to a diverse and significant number of users, is an integral part of the vision of health care reform. A complex modern society cannot elevate each person's interest in privacy above other societal interests."[1] We can easily deceive ourselves, however, into thinking that our data gathering will be used only for the good of the individual and society. Without appropriate safeguards, the collection of medical data could turn into medical surveillance. If people perceive their records as semipublic and the use of health care services as a threat to personal privacy, patients might forgo treatment, avoid the network by paying out of pocket, or seek alternative therapies.

Conclusion

Individuals have the right to expect, and the health care system has the obligation to provide, assurances that records will be kept confidential and maintained in a secure system. The computerization of health records and involvement of private and government health insurance plans raise serious questions about easy access to records and the semipublic nature of medical records. Legislation will address some of these concerns. We cannot be paralyzed by potential abuses related to the electronic medical record, but we should not be naive about the challenges. We must use the computer responsibly with the goals of improving the quality of care and protecting patient privacy.

Note

1. L. Gostin, "Health Information Privacy," *Cornell Law Review* 80 (1995), 515.

Chapter 22 _____

CPR and DNR Revisited

About sixty years ago, when a person's heart stopped beating and the lungs stopped breathing, the person was declared dead. Through a series of experiments in the 1940s, however, researchers discovered that the heart could be resuscitated through drugs and electrical stimulation. In 1960 research demonstrated that circulation also could be restored by external cardiac massage. At first emergency cardiac resuscitation was used mainly in recovery rooms at hospitals and by persons called upon to give emergency medical care—such as lifeguards, police, firefighters, and ambulance personnel. In the 1970s and 1980s hospitals and long-term care centers developed policies that mandated resuscitation efforts—cardiopulmonary resuscitation (CPR)—for all patients who suffered cardiac arrest. Experience quickly demonstrated, however, that not all persons suffering cardiac arrest in health care facilities would benefit from CPR. In an effort to designate in advance patients who would not benefit from CPR or who did not want this form of therapy, "Do Not Resuscitate" (DNR) orders were developed in many health care facilities. In spite of the frequent use of CPR and the frequent issuance of DNR orders, several ethical issues continue to occur in hospitals and long-term care facilities with regard to cardiopulmonary resuscitation.

Principles

Cardiac arrest occurs at some point in the dying process of every person, whatever the underlying cause of death. Hence, the decision of whether to attempt resuscitation is potentially relevant for all patients. In theory, CPR for cardiac arrest is a multi-step process. Usually it includes chest compression, administration of various medications, electrical shocks to restart the heart, placement of a breathing tube (intubation), and use of a breathing machine (ventilator). In practice, however, the medical team conducting CPR will not wait to see if the initial steps are successful before beginning more aggressive procedures.

Thus, CPR is usually envisioned as a single therapy aimed at restoring cardiopulmonary function. As such, it may be evaluated ethically like other life-prolonging therapies. The essential ethical question for its use is, Will it benefit the overall well-being of the patient?

Patient well-being is discerned by considering more than the patient's physiological function. Keeping the patient alive is not the ultimate criterion for ethical medical care; the social and creative function of the patient must also be considered. Specifically, overall patient benefit may be discerned by asking two questions: Does the life-prolonging therapy impose a grave burden on the patient? Is the therapy ineffective insofar as the overall well-being of the patient is concerned? If either of these questions is answered affirmatively, there is no ethical imperative to utilize the therapy in question.

Discussion

Although the general principles for use of CPR are not difficult to understand, over the years the application of these principles has raised several ethical questions. Who should be considered an apt patient for CPR? For whom should DNR orders be written? Studies demonstrate that severely debilitated patients—for example, those suffering from cancer or sepsis—seldom recover cardiopulmonary function after CPR. Even when severely debilitated patients have been resuscitated, some have survived in a persistent vegetative state. Many of those who did recover some degree of cognitive-affective function died of other causes before leaving the hospital.

To withhold CPR from a patient through a DNR order, it must be determined in advance that attempts at resuscitation would either impose a grave burden on the patient or be ineffective therapy insofar as the overall well-being of the patient is concerned. When would CPR be considered a grave burden in relation to the benefit it might bring? In this regard, several people mention the broken bones and bruises that may result from the various steps in the resuscitative process. Although some physical injury may result from CPR, in most cases withholding it on the grounds of physical burden would not be reasonable if weighed against the benefit of prolonged life. Perhaps a patient with severe osteoporosis would suffer serious injury from CPR that would not be offset by the benefits, but it is not immediately evident that others would experience the same burden.

When assessing grave burden, other sources of burden besides physiological suffering should be considered. For example, the economic, social, and spiritual effects of the therapy must also be evaluated. The President's Commission on Ethics in Medicine opined that resuscitation efforts usually provide benefits that justify their costs. In itself CPR would not seem to impose a social or spiritual burden on the patient or the family, unless it could be foreseen that resuscitation would result in a respirator-dependent condition. If this outcome were predicted, living in this condition might be considered too burdensome, and a request for a DNR order might be in order.

Would CPR ever be *ineffective* therapy insofar as a patient's well-being is concerned? Would CPR be effective therapy for a person in a persistent vegetative state, or for a person in a seriously demented condition? Would CPR benefit patients with end-stage diseases, such as cancer of the lungs or pancreas, if it would prolong their lives for only a few days? When a determination is made that CPR would be ineffective, it is an admission that this therapy is not conducive to the overall well-being of the patient—either because it is unlikely to benefit the patient (which should be demonstrated through clinical research) or because it will not benefit the patient even if it does work. Declaring a therapy to be ineffective is an admission that science and medicine are unable to benefit the patient. Declaring a therapy to be ineffective is not the same as saying the therapy will not prolong life.

Who decides whether CPR will be beneficial for the overall well-being of the patient? Who is the person responsible for determining that a DNR order will be issued because CPR will impose a grave burden or be ineffective? For many years, this decision was considered to be the prerogative of the competent patient or a proxy (if the patient were incapable of making the health care decisions). As evidence proving the ineffectiveness of CPR for some patients became more extensive, however, it was suggested that an attending physician could make this decision unilaterally without communicating it to the patient or proxy. Thus, an attending physician could determine that CPR was not an apt therapy for certain patients, just as an attending physician can determine that laetrile is not fitting therapy for reversing the growth of cancer cells. In certain circumstances physicians should make a decision that CPR is not an effective therapy. This kind of judgment is well within the ambit of ethical medicine. Because CPR is considered a standard therapy, however, this decision should be communicated to the patient or proxy. Writing a DNR without communicating this decision to patients or their proxies would violate their moral right to informed consent.

In the everyday practice, the "slow code," or "Hollywood code," is sometimes in evidence. This practice is characterized by "going through the motions," a decision having been made in advance by caregivers that the patient will not benefit from CPR, although no one has had the courage to write the DNR order. Similar to this approach is the predetermined decision to utilize only part of the CPR procedures—to withhold electrical shock and intubation if less aggressive steps do not restore cardiopulmonary function. The many steps of CPR have one goal: to restore cardiopulmonary function. Half-hearted efforts to achieve this goal would be unethical. If the therapy is judged likely to be effective, it should be utilized in a way that will ensure its success. Stopping CPR halfway through the process is simply another manner of going through the motions.

Conclusion

Does writing a DNR order necessarily imply that the patient should have all life-prolonging therapy withdrawn? In general, the answer to this question is no. Each life-prolonging therapy should be judged on its own merits. The medical indications that would justify withholding CPR may discourage the use of other therapies. Hence, if a DNR is written for an unconscious patient with end-stage disease, an evaluation of all life-prolonging therapy is in order.

Chapter 23 _____

Living Will and Durable Power of Attorney

In recent years, several prominent court cases have been concerned with the removal of life support from people no longer able to make medical decisions for themselves. As people discuss the Quinlan, Brophy, O'Connor, Cruzan, Busalacchi, and Finn cases, they affirm the desire to avoid such disputes if they were ever in the same condition. To facilitate the desire to avoid unwanted therapy and doubt concerning preferred treatment when patients are in danger of death, many states have approved the use of living wills (LW) and durable powers of attorney (DPA) for health affairs. Both documents allow still-competent persons to express the way they would like medical care to be rendered when they are incapacitated—that is, no longer capable of medical decision making. Usually, the decision that a person is incapacitated is made by one or two physicians.

These documents exonerate the persons who implement them from any civil or criminal liability. In general, the LW is implemented by an attending physician, and the DPA is implemented by a proxy, known as the agent or attorney-in-fact. The LW is to be implemented when death threatens and the person is incapable of medical decision making. The DPA is implemented as soon as the person becomes incapable of medical decision making; it is operative regardless of whether death threatens. Although both documents are inherently ethical, they are often ineffective in accomplishing the goals that people have in mind when they sign them. This chapter seeks to explain the difficulties involved in the use of both documents and offers some suggestions that may alleviate the difficulties.

Difficulties

One serious difficulty arises because many people, especially physicians who have fear of malpractice litigation, believe that life support may not be withheld or removed if a patient has not signed an LW or DPA. Even if a patient has not executed an LW or DPA, however, the ethical right to withhold or remove life support that is no longer beneficial is still present. In other words, although a clearly written LW or DPA may facilitate the removal of life support, if a document of this nature has not been executed by the patient the family still has a moral right to make decisions for the incapacitated person. We receive the ethical responsibility to make decisions concerning our own health care and the health care of our incapacitated loved ones from our nature as human beings, not from positive civil law. Court decisions and state laws may recognize and structure our ethical decision-making rights, but they do not create these rights. Hence, the LW and DPA may facilitate good decision making, but they do not create the moral power to make such decisions.

A second difficulty often arises because state laws usually contain model forms for people to sign while still competent. The wording of these model forms often gives rise to ambiguity and ethical questions. When Sam, a young man in a coma as a result of an automobile accident, was brought to the emergency room, his family told the trauma surgeons that Sam had stated that he never wanted a respirator or artificial hydration and nutrition to be used in his behalf. Moreover, they had a DPA that expressed this wish on Sam's part. The physicians countered by saying that "If we don't use these life supports Sam will die, and we have seen people in worse conditions eventually walk out of here." After some persuasion, the family consented to the use of a ventilator as well as artificial hydration and nutrition. The happy ending of the story is that Sam did recover and walked out of a rehabilitation center four months later. The essential issue in this case, however, is not the success of the therapy; it is the nature of the decision that must be made when caring for seriously debilitated persons. Certainly, an attorney-in-fact has the right to request removal of life support that is a grave burden or ineffective. Therapy cannot be judged to be a grave burden or ineffective, however, unless the medical condition of the patient and the hope for recovery (diagnosis and prognosis) are known. Supplying this information is the responsibility of the physician.

As a result of ambiguous language, the LWs have been ineffective and have been supplanted in many states by DPAs for health affairs. Through a DPA the agent usually is given the power to make all health care decisions for the now-incapacitated person, even if the patient is not in a terminal condition. In some states confinement to a mental institution or use of electroconvulsive therapy requires a court order in addition to a decision by the agent.

The greatest potential difficulty of a DPA is in language indicating that the agent will make health care decisions in accord with the values and principles that the patient would follow if he or she were capable of decision making. This provision presupposes that the person making the DPA has thought through his or her desires and communicated them to the agent. Just as a marriage license does not ensure the existence of marital love, however, a DPA does not ensure that the proper communication has taken place.

Clearly, the agent is given extensive powers of decision making through the DPA. What about the responsibilities of the physician? Physicians are also patient advocates, not blind servants of surrogate decision makers. Ethical health care for incapacitated patients with DPAs will still require cooperation between physicians and surrogates. Although some physicians have welcomed the DPA because it frees them from legal liability and enables them to work with a definite person as surrogate, it does not free them from ethical responsibilities. Physicians must still offer and implement plans for medical treatment in accord with the overall well-being of the patient.

Solutions

Although there are no easy solutions to the aforementioned difficulties, the following suggestions may be of some help.

- Medical decisions may be made for incapacitated patients even if they have not executed an LW or DPA. These decisions should be made by loved ones in collaboration with the attending physician using ethical norms followed for centuries: "If able to make a decision, what would mom or dad want in these circumstances?"
- Because the interpretation of an LW is sometimes ambiguous, utilize a DPA to allow it to fulfill the goals of the LW. Hence, state explicitly that the DPA will be effective at all times—even as death approaches.
- Be sure to discuss your desires and values with the person designated as agent. In this discussion focus on the mental and physical functions you consider necessary for a meaningful life; that is, point out the impairments and disabilities that would justify withholding or removing life support. For example, if you have advanced Alzheimer's disease, do you wish to be treated for pneumonia? If you have not thought through your values and desires, perhaps you would ask your proxy to act in accord with the teaching of your church with regard to the use and removal of life support.
- Realize that you can state reservations in your DPA. For example, will you allow your agent to commit you to a mental institution without a court order?

- Avoid mentioning specific medical treatments that you wish excluded in the event you are incapacitated. The very therapy you exclude (e.g. artificial hydration and nutrition) may be the therapy that will restore you to decision-making capacity. Instead, encourage life support, but include the desire to have it removed if it does not restore function that would be essential for you to pursue the purpose of life.
- If you have a physician that you see consistently, give her or him a copy of your DPA and explain the preferences you have for therapy as death approaches.

Conclusion

The ethical norms for medical care and life-prolonging therapy are clear; life should be prolonged unless the therapy to prolong life imposes a grave burden or is ineffective insofar as the overall well-being of the patient is concerned. Used wisely, a DPA follows these norms. Moreover, it can keep decision making out of the legal forum and in the family forum— where it belongs.

Chapter 24 _____

The Patient Self-Determination Act (PSDA)

The Patient Self-Determination Act (PSDA), which went into effect in December 1991, has changed considerably the manner in which health care facilities offer patient care. The overall purpose of the Act is to increase the use of advance directives for health care. This chapter considers briefly the main provisions of the PSDA and more extensively some ethical issues to which the legislation may give rise.

Principles

The main provisions of the PSDA affecting health care facilities and physicians are as follows:

1. Every health care facility that receives Medicare or Medicaid funding from the federal government must give to each incoming patient a statement of rights with regard to making health care decisions. Thus, the bill applies to hospitals, nursing homes, home health agencies, hospice programs, and HMOs. The statement of rights will be derived from the law and court decisions of the state in which the facility is located.

2. The health care facility also must ask patients if they have advance directives. If a person has made an advance directive, this fact must be documented in the medical record. The simplest way to fulfill this stipulation may be to place a copy of the advance directive in the patient's chart. If the patient has not executed an advance directive, this fact also must be documented—although health care may not be withheld for that reason.

3. The facility must also give the patient an explanation of its own policy with regard to advance directives. If the provisions of the patient's advance directive violate the policies of the facility, the patient must be informed that some stipulations of the advance directive will not be honored. For example, if an advance directive calls for physician-assisted euthanasia, facilities that oppose such a practice should have a statement prepared in advance that explains that advance directives containing such requests will not be honored.

4. The health care facility must "ensure compliance with the requirements of state law." For this purpose, the facility has the duty to provide education programs for staff members and the community regarding advance directives and their meaning. Clearly, physicians and other health care professionals will need instructions concerning effective implementation of advance directives.

At least three significant ethical issues may arise as the result of this legislation:

- If they have not done so already, some patients may wish to execute advance directives at the time of admission to the health care facility. Because of the tension, anxiety, and depression many people experience when they are admitted to a nursing home, hospital, or hospice program, this is a poor time to make decisions concerning future health care. Moreover, advance directives should be made after prudent reflection and from a perspective of faith. Allowing patients to prepare hurried advance directives fosters the depersonalization of medicine. In general, then, for the benefit of all concerned parties, advance directives should be executed well before patients are admitted to health care facilities. If a patient has not executed an advance directive and wishes to do so at the time of admission, the facility should attempt to persuade the person to delay the process. If a patient insists on executing a directive at the time of admission, the facility should provide counseling in regard to the meaning and effects of the document.

- Because an advance directive is such an important document, the person who will make health care decisions for an incapacitated person should know the goals and wishes of the person who has executed the document. Often, communication between the person who executes the advance directive and the person who will ensure compliance with it is weak or nonexistent. How can one act as a reputable agent for another unless the proxy is able to "stand in the shoes" of the patient? Studies show that the decisions of proxies are inaccurate if effective communication has not taken place. If communication between patients and the persons who will become their agents is nonexistent or weak, the process of decision making may become a legalistic farce.

- The need for communication between patient and proxy is also obvious if advance directives have not been executed. Legislation authorizing advance directives does not create the right of proxy decision making. Rather, such legislation merely regulates this proxy decision making and seeks to make the exercise of this right more effective. The proxy for a person who has not executed an advance directive usually will be a family member. Unless some serious conversation has taken place concerning the wishes of the patient, the proxy will be left without any objective evidence for decision making. The use of artificial nutrition and hydration, for example, should be discussed explicitly. People with a living faith will do well to discuss the implications of their faith with family members so that decisions concerning the prolongation of life will be formulated in accord with their religious beliefs.

Conclusion

Although an advance directive is a useful and beneficial method of exercising one's natural right to make decisions concerning health care, the sledgehammer approach of the PSDA may cause more problems than it solves. Clearly, medical care should be withheld and life support should be removed if they are not beneficial for the patient. Deciding what is beneficial, however, is an act of love on the part of the proxy and an act of advocacy on the part of the physician. Love and advocacy are frustrated unless adequate communication and empathy precede medical decision making.

Chapter 25

Advance Directives Revisited

A recent study by Joan Teno and Joanne Lynn at the George Washington University Center to Improve Care for the Dying and seven other medical centers fuels ongoing concerns about the effectiveness of advance directives in health care.[1] The results reveal that only 14 percent of 4,804 terminally ill patients had written medical directives. Fewer than 30 of these 569 documents contained specific instructions about the use of life-sustaining treatment, and only 22 directives matched the patient's actual situation. Even when specific instructions were present, care was inconsistent with those instructions in half of the cases. Moreover, increasing the documentation of advance directives was not associated with a reduction in hospital resource use. These findings suggest that advance directives accomplish little on their own.

Advance directives have been praised for years as ethical instruments that enhance individual autonomy, facilitate decision making, and eliminate ineffective care at the end of life. The empirical evidence, however, seems to refute these claims. Documents that focus primarily on treatment interventions rarely guide medical decision making beyond naming a health care proxy or documenting general preferences. Despite intense publicity and encouragement to the public to complete medical directives, few dying patients have them; when they do, the documents make little or no difference in medical care. Why haven't advance directives lived up to their early promise of enabling patient choice? Are there more effective ways to enhance dialogue and design care that include, but are not limited to, life-sustaining treatments?

The Promise of Advance Directives

Over the past two decades, every state has provided mechanisms for people to declare what treatment they want to forego if they are unable to make decisions about health care, to name a proxy who would make such decisions, or both. Since December 1991, the federal Patient Self-Determination Act (PSDA) has required that health care providers inform adult patients upon admission of their rights under state laws to participate in decisions about medical treatment. An additional intent of the PSDA was to educate the public about living wills and health care powers of attorney. In part, the fear of being at the mercy of medical and legal paternalism, as well as the hope of saving resources at the end of life, stimulated the PSDA. The PSDA was aimed at giving patients legitimate choice and voice regarding end-of-life decisions.

There would seem to be few reasons to quibble with such intentions. As originally conceived, advance directives had much to recommend them. They had the potential to encourage patients to reflect on end-of life issues, allow patients to share their treatment preferences and goals with those who would care for them at the end of life, and help resolve some fears about ineffective or overly burdensome life-sustaining treatment. Ideally, these documents would give a degree of legal protection to physicians and health care institutions and thus foster physician-patient communication. Health care directives would also make it easier for relatives to know the person's wishes and to feel comfortable making decisions on behalf of their loved ones. All of these advantages, however, imply leadership by health care professionals and facilities to inform, discuss, and ultimately advise patients on end-of-life treatment interventions.

The Reality of Advance Directives

The changing nature of the physician-patient relationship has affected the use of advance directives. Increasingly, health care professionals are regarded as entrepreneurs or contractors, and patients are regarded as customers or consumers. In this environment, physicians and health care facilities can use an advance directive as an excuse not to communicate with patients and their families. They can justify this abrogation of responsibility by invoking the claim of respect for patient autonomy. If physicians and patients are viewed as "equal contractors," and patients employ their physicians for specific technical acts of healing, adhering blindly to advance directives about specific treatment interventions makes sense. Respect for patient autonomy, however, implies more rather than less physician involvement; it requires that physicians genuinely seek to remain in dialogue with patients and their families. True autonomy implies a freedom of choice that is possible only when patients, their loved ones, and physicians act jointly in addressing immediate and ultimate goals.

The vexing reality is that living wills and health care powers of attorney are still relatively rare. Although public opinion polls consistently show support for the use of advance directives, few people actually complete them. In December 1993, the U.S. Department of Health and Human Services conducted a comprehensive review at seventy-two facilities (twenty-four each of hospitals, nursing facilities, and home health agencies) in six states. Only 21 percent of the patients in these facilities had advance directives. People without advance directives claimed their families would know what they would want. Of those with advance directives, slightly more than half actually had copies in the medical chart. The lack of clear and consistent documentation in patients' charts increased the possibility that their treatment wishes would not be followed. Facilities reported that patient understanding often was very poor on admission because of anxiety surrounding their health condition and the number of papers presented to them. These findings support the suggestion that the provision of information should begin well *before* the patient is admitted to a facility.

A Change in Focus: Advance Care Planning

Obviously, advance directives do not solve all problems. Some people have proposed advance care planning as an alternative. A study in the October 1997 *Annals of Internal Medicine* explores this process of helping patients and families think through and communicate the overall goals of care—which include, but are not limited to, decisions about life-sustaining treatments. Advance care planning considers how the goals of medical care change in different situations. There are several questions that physicians, patients, and families should discuss to clarify health care goals and preferences. Who should speak on your behalf if you are so sick that you cannot speak for yourself? If you became seriously ill today, what should be the goals of your medical care? What are the factors that influence your choices? If you were facing a life-threatening event, are there circumstances under which all you would want is to be kept comfortable? What are these circumstances? Are there any life-sustaining treatments you know you would not want under any circumstances? What is it about these treatments that makes them undesirable? Are there any life-sustaining treatments you know you would want regardless of the situation? Why would you want these treatments? What are your fears and concerns about the way that you might die? In the event you were dying, where would you want to receive care? Finally, should your current preferences be strictly applied to future situations, or should they serve as a guide for your proxy decision makers?

Conclusion

Advance directives serve a limited purpose when they address treatment interventions only at the end of life. Patients may not fully understand treatments and outcomes, or they may have difficulty formulating and expressing preferences about future situations. Patients may also change their minds when faced with the actual decision to forego life-sustaining treatment. Advance care planning will not solve all these problems; it still involves a commitment of time and requires a relationship based on trust and respect. It may help assure, however, that personal and professional caregivers understand the patient's moral convictions and attitudes toward healing and dying, as well as their preferences regarding life-sustaining treatment.

Note

1. Joan Teno and Joanne Lyn, "Measuring Quality of Care at the End of Life." *Journal of the American Geriatrics Society* 45 (April 1997): 399–406, 500–507, 508–12.

Part Three

Use and Removal of Life Support

Chapter 26

Ordinary and Extraordinary Means

When discussing the care of a dying patient, people often use the terms *ordinary* and *extraordinary* means as though they solve all ethical questions. Closer analysis often reveals, however, that these terms do not lead to clear solutions. Are the terms useful or meaningful in ethical discourse? They can be, if a few distinctions are kept in mind.

Principles

Clearly, physicians and ethicists approach the dying patient with different emphases: The ethicist is more concerned with how the person dies, whereas the physician is more concerned with how to prolong life. When particular ethical cases are being decided, there need not be any radical disagreement between physicians and ethicists if three truths are clearly distinguished:

1. Physicians and moralists often use the terms "ordinary means" and "extraordinary means" with different connotations.
2. Although the physician has the expertise and the right to make decisions concerning the usefulness of medical effects of particular means, the patient (or the patient's family) has the right to determine whether a particular means is ordinary or extraordinary from an ethical point of view.
3. If the means are determined from an ethical point of view to be ordinary, they must be employed; if they are determined to be extraordinary, they may or may not be employed—the decision being

made by the patient (or the family) in consultation with the physician (although ordinary care should continue).

Discussion

Physicians often use the term "ordinary means" to describe an accepted or standard medical procedure. A procedure that is new and untested or still in the experimental stage is called *extraordinary* or *heroic*. Thus, from the physician's point of view, most means could be classified as ordinary or extraordinary without any reference to a patient. From a medical perspective, then, a respirator, tube feeding, or use of an artificial heart was at one time extraordinary but became ordinary by reason of effectiveness and acceptability.

The ethicist, on the other hand, sees these terms in a different light. For the ethicist, ordinary and extraordinary means have no meaning unless the patient's condition is known. For example, one cannot designate a respirator or tube feeding as ordinary or extraordinary from an ethical perspective unless the patient's diagnosis and prognosis are known. The ethicist assumes that a person has a need or obligation to prolong human life but that there are limits to this need or obligation. One obvious limit is that one need not do something useless to prolong life. Thus, if a patient dying of cancer contracts pneumonia, it is generally agreed that the patient may refuse treatment for pneumonia if his or her life would not be prolonged for a significant time. One need not seek all possible cures for a fatal condition if there is little hope that any of them would be successful.

Another limit to the obligation to prolong life occurs when the means to prolong life would involve a grave burden to the person insofar as the more important values of life are concerned. For example, classical ethicists maintained that a surgical procedure might be declared extraordinary because of the concomitant burden it might involve. Today we might declare a quadruple amputation extraordinary from an ethical perspective— not because of the actual pain of the surgery but because of the burden that life in this condition might impose on the person.

In maintaining that one is free to make a judgment not to prolong life because a grave burden would result, even though prolonging life is possible, we are affirming that although human life is a great good, it is not the greatest good. This affirmation is the practical meaning of the word *burden:* making it difficult for one to attain the purpose of life.

Ethically speaking, then, ordinary means of preserving life are medicines, treatments, and operations that offer a reasonable hope of benefit for the patient and can be obtained or used without excessive expense, pain, or burden. Extraordinary means are medicines, treatments, and operations that cannot be used or obtained without excessive expense, pain, or other burden or do not offer a reasonable hope of benefit.

Some ethicists maintain that the terms *ordinary* and *extraordinary* are inadequate for the decision-making task in ethics. The theoretical difficulties could be eliminated if the first question is not, Is this means ordinary or extraordinary? but, Is there an obligation to prolong life? Thus, the patient's condition and value system must first be discerned. If the answer to this latter question is affirmative, the medical means necessary to prolong life are ordinary means from an ethical perspective. If there is no obligation to prolong life, then only procedures that will keep the patient comfortable are ordinary means; all other means are extraordinary from an ethical perspective.

The practical difficulties in applying the distinction between ordinary and extraordinary means to prolong life will always remain. Determining whether it is time to allow oneself to die—or to allow another to die—will always be a complex decision for a compassionate person, especially if the decision involves discontinuing a means already in use. This difficulty is evidenced excruciatingly in the case of newborns with birth defects. The difficulties do not destroy the use of the distinction, however.

Clearly, the physician is responsible for deciding which therapies are ordinary and which are extraordinary, but who is responsible for deciding this matter from the ethical perspective? The physician must be involved in the decision because the diagnosis and prognosis will depend mainly on his or her science and skill, but the patient has the ultimate responsibility for making this decision. The patient retains this responsibility not only because he or she has the right to determine which values will be pursued but because only the patient knows the other circumstances—for example, the pain, expense, or inconvenience involved in a particular therapy—that must be considered in making the ethical decision.

Conclusion

More difficult problems arise when the patient is incompetent and cannot make the ethical decision. Although some people would refer all such decisions to the courts, the courts should be consulted only when a manifest injustice might be inflicted on an incompetent patient. More often, the family or spouse should decide for the incompetent patient for two reasons: they love the patient and will decide what is best for the person, and they know the patient's mind and should be able to request what he or she would want. Physicians and family members should cooperate in the decision-making process. Neither group should assert an adversarial position; both groups should seek to make decisions that are beneficial for the patient.

Chapter 27

Ethical Criteria for Removing Life Support

Christine Busalacchi was injured in an automobile accident in 1987. After a series of acute-care interventions were unsuccessful, she was diagnosed as being in a persistent vegetative state (PVS). Because of the PVS condition, she was unable to eat or swallow. This fatal pathology was circumvented through medically assisted hydration and nutrition. Six years after the accident, when the courts in Missouri finally determined that her medical care should be under the direction of her father, a controversy arose concerning the ethics of removing life support from a person in a persistent vegetative state. Specifically, the question of removing artificial hydration and nutrition from Christine was debated on television, in the press, and among health care personnel. Emotion and pietistic assumptions more often than sound ethical reasoning seemed to prompt most statements concerning Christine's care. In an effort to clarify the proper care of persons in a PVS, this chapter considers the facts and questions that are relevant for an ethical withdrawal of life support.

Principles

When considering the use or removal of life support, the first relevant fact concerns the existence of a fatal pathology. A fatal pathology is an illness, disease, or bodily condition that will cause the death of a person if the effects of the pathology are not circumvented or alleviated. Examples of fatal pathologies are diabetes, cancer, or end-stage renal disease. If a fatal pathology is present, the question arises: Should attempts be made to remove, circumvent, or alleviate the pathology through medical therapy? Or should nature be allowed to take its course, thus allowing the person to die of the existing pathology? Should diabetes be circumvented through the use of insulin? Should attempts be made to remove the cancer through surgery? Should attempts be made to alleviate the end-stage renal disease through hemodialysis? Usually, people wish to combat fatal pathologies by means of medical therapy. They opt for insulin, surgery, or hemodialysis if their lives are threatened.

In most cases, there is an ethical conviction as well as a natural intuition to preserve life through medical therapy because it enables one to strive for the important goods of life. What are these important goods? In general, the important goods are preserving life, seeking the truth, loving our families, generating and nurturing future generations, and forming communities with other people. In addition to these goods, each one of us has particular goods that are important to our sense of purpose and well-being.

In some situations however, extending life through medical therapy does not enable the patient to strive for the important goods of life—or, if it does, the therapy imposes a burden that makes striving for the goods of life too difficult. To be more specific, because of the condition of the patient, medical therapy may be either ineffective—making it impossible for the person to pursue the important goods of life—or it may impose an excessive burden, making it too difficult for the person to strive for important goods of life. One situation in which medical therapy usually is ineffective occurs when the patient's death is imminent and unavoidable. Hence, a conscious patient who is severely debilitated as a result of pathologies in many organs may request removal of a respirator because continued existence in this condition will not allow her or him to pursue any of the goods of life. Moreover, the same decision to remove life support may be made by family members for an incapacitated loved one, if the hope that the patient will recover consciousness is slight and death is imminent and unavoidable.

Another condition that renders medical therapy ineffective is the persistent vegetative state (PVS). Because of a dysfunctional cerebral cortex, persons in this condition can never again strive for the goods of life that we identify with creative (or spiritual) human function. Their cognitive-affective function is nonexistent and cannot be restored. Thus, they do not have the power to think, love, relate to others, or demonstrate care and compassion—nor can these powers ever be regained. In addition, because of damage to the cerebral cortex, persons in PVS are unable to eat, chew, and swallow. This pathology can be circumvented by means of medically assisted hydration and nutrition. Does use of this medical therapy benefit the patient? Does prolonging physiological function, with the realization that the patient will be unable to strive for most of the important goods of life, mandate continued medical intervention? Simply because a person in a PVS may be kept alive does not indicate that the person must be kept alive. Removing life support from persons in PVS is not euthanasia because it neither induces a new cause of death nor implies the intention of killing the patient.

Medical therapy that imposes an excessive burden for a patient may also be discontinued. An excessive burden may affect a patient's ability to strive for a physiological good, a social good, or a spiritual good that is very important to the patient. The excessive burden under consideration need not be directly associated with the therapy, though it often results from the use of the therapy. Examples of excessive burden that impede the pursuit of more important human goods occur frequently. A patient with end-stage renal disease opts for discontinuing dialysis because he is bedridden and lacks energy to relate to others or care for himself. The father of a family refuses to have surgery because it would involve selling the family home or expending funds designated for the education of his children. A Jehovah's Witness refuses a life-prolonging blood transfusion because she believes receiving blood transfusions is a serious sin.

Discussion

The question concerning excessive burden is posed after a decision is made that the therapy is effective. Hence, there are two distinct criteria that come into consideration after the existence of a fatal pathology has been medically ascertained: Is the therapy effective? If the therapy is effective, does it impose an excessive burden now or in the future? Both of these criteria require an evaluation of the patient's ability to strive for the goods of life. In some situations, medical therapy will not enable the person to strive for the goods of life. Such therapy would be ineffective. In some conditions, medical therapy would enable a person to continue striving for the goods of life, but the therapy would also impose burdens that would make striving for the goods of life very difficult. Such therapy would be an excessive burden.

Determining whether therapy is ineffective depends on objective evidence more than determining excessive burden does. Agreement on the condition that will lead to imminent and unavoidable death or the inability to regain cognitive-affective function may be reached by objective medical diagnosis. Determining excessive burden is much more subjective, however. Two people may react differently to the burden of prolonged dialysis treatment. Hence, when people are unable to consent for themselves, it is important to have some idea of how they would evaluate the burden if they were able. Finally, because we are social beings, whether patients decide for themselves or through proxies, evaluation of burden must take into consideration the burden placed on the family and community.

One more question is relevant in considering the removal of life support: What is the intention of the people removing the life support? Clearly, actions that are morally good in themselves may be performed with bad intentions. A person may give money to the poor simply to enhance his or her reputation. Thus, even an external act of charity can be perverted by a bad intention.

Many people believe that if life support is removed because it is ineffective or because it imposes an excessive burden, the intention of the family or medical team is to cause the death of the patient. If this were the intention of the people removing life support, it would be unethical. Usually, however, when life support is removed because it is ineffective, the intention of the family and medical team is to cease doing something futile. When life support is removed because it imposes an excessive burden, the intention is to remove some form of physiological, social, or spiritual burden from the patient. When people remove life support from a loved one because it is ineffective or a serious burden, they often express relief or even joy. Thus, we hear: "Mom has died but she is better off," "Dad's death was a blessing." What people are expressing through these words is relief and joy that the burden has been removed, not joy and relief that mom or dad is dead. If the ineffective or burdensome therapy could be removed without the ensuing death of mom or dad, loving children would remove the therapy in a manner that would prolong life. Given the realities of life, however, when removing life support becomes ethically necessary, the death of the loved one usually follows as an act of nature. It is not desired or intended by the people removing the life support.

Conclusion

Four questions summarize the ethical process that should be followed when removing life support:

1. Is a fatal pathology present in the body of the patient?
2. Does resisting the fatal pathology involve effective or ineffective therapy?
3. If the therapy is effective, does the therapy impose an excessive burden?
4. What is the intention of the persons who are deciding whether to remove life support?

The ethical process described above is based on a vision of human life as a quest for goods that fulfill the innate and acquired needs of the person. Human life is a dynamic process that involves fulfilling interrelated needs through the pursuit of goods. The purpose of medical therapy is to enable a person to fulfill needs by pursuing goods. Medical therapy often accomplishes this goal. When medical therapy does not enable a person with a fatal pathology to pursue the goods of life or makes this pursuit too burdensome, however, the medical therapy may be withheld or withdrawn, even though death would result.

Chapter 28 _____

Withholding and Withdrawing Life Support

In 1983 the President's Commission on Ethics in Health Care rejected the principle that stopping (withdrawing) a treatment is morally more serious than not starting (withholding) it.[1] In 1989 the American Academy of Neurology, in its commentary on the treatment of patients in a persistent vegetative state, avowed that "the view that there is a major medical or ethical distinction between the withholding and withdrawal of medical treatment belies common sense and good medical practice. . . ."[2] Nevertheless, in the world of clinical medicine, confusion remains in regard to this issue, sometimes with tragic consequences. For example, in 1988 Sammy Linares, a six-month-old baby, aspirated a balloon and eventually lapsed into a persistent vegetative state. The father of the child asked that treatment be discontinued and the child be allowed to die. The hospital lawyer insisted that although withholding treatment would be all right, removing treatment constituted killing the child. Eventually the father removed the child from the ventilator at gunpoint. This tragic story suggests that a need exists to review the distinctions between withholding and withdrawing treatment and evaluate whether such distinctions have any ethical significance.

Principles

Clearly, a physical distinction exists between not starting and discontinuing treatment. One is an action of omission, the other of commission. In many minds, this physical distinction implies an ethical distinction as well. Specifically, some people contend that withholding treatment merely allows nature to run its course, whereas withdrawing treatment seems to introduce a new cause of death and kills the patient. The existential emotional and psychological reactions people have to removing treatment reinforce this ethical distinction. Does the ethical distinction between withdrawing and withholding treatment follow from the physical and emotional distinctions?

Proper assessment of the moral significance of the action requires an examination of the intentions of the action. When one appropriately withdraws treatment from a patient, one intends to avoid a treatment that has become overly burdensome or now is judged to be ineffective. In withholding treatment, similar intentions are involved—except that one initially assumes that the treatment will be too burdensome or ineffective without a trial course. In both cases, one does not intend death but instead chooses no longer to circumvent an existing fatal pathology because therapy no longer benefits the patient. Consequently, on the level of intention, withdrawing and withholding treatment are ethically the same.

In this analysis, the underlying intention determines the ethical nature of the action. As the President's Commission explained, the distinction between omission and commission is ethically unimportant, albeit emotionally significant. From this viewpoint, withholding treatment can be equally inappropriate as withdrawing it if one in fact has an obligation to supply treatment.

In addition, making an ethical distinction between withholding and withdrawing treatment threatens to compromise patient care in two ways. First, such an ethical distinction implies that once a caregiver starts a treatment, it cannot be removed or that removal requires greater justification.

The paradigmatic case of Nancy Beth Cruzan illustrates the inappropriate patient care that results from such faulty ethical analysis. Of greater concern is that because of the issues arising in the Cruzan scenario, caregivers may withhold potentially beneficial care out of fear that once started, treatment could not be removed even if the expected benefit did not result. Second, patient autonomy and the goals of informed consent may be violated as patients receive treatments that they (or their surrogates) may not desire, which can result in burdens (emotional, physical, financial) for the patient, family, and society.

Discussion and Applications

To provide a practical solution to this problem, caregivers may offer a treatment on a trial basis with the explicit understanding that if the treatment is ineffective or too burdensome, it can be discontinued. This approach obviates the possibility of wrongly withholding a beneficial treatment out of fear of not being able to remove it, and it promotes legitimate patient autonomy. When a treatment's efficacy is unclear, one requires greater justification to withhold treatment than to withdraw it because treatment efficacy cannot be determined until a trial is completed. This trial-basis approach may prevent situations wherein patients (or most likely surrogates) request the indefinite continuation of medically futile treatments.

Nevertheless, despite the reasonableness of this approach, caregivers should recognize and anticipate the emotional responses that some people have to withdrawing treatment. The first is the misconception over culpability resulting from withdrawing versus withholding treatment. Second, caregivers may be more reluctant to withdraw treatment because of the investment (money, time, energy) that has been made in the patient. Continuing to offer ineffective treatment will not make previous treatment worthwhile, however, and it can harm the patient's well-being. Third, caregivers and family members may feel that in withdrawing treatment, they are abandoning or giving up on the patient. Proper ongoing comfort care can help alleviate such misgivings about abandonment. Finally, fearing the perception by others that some inappropriate criterion precipitated their decision to remove treatment, caregivers may make a psychological distinction between withholding and withdrawing treatment. Although caregivers should be sensitive to the possibility that they are removing treatment for inappropriate reasons, that awareness should not prevent them from withdrawing treatment for sound ethical and medical reasons.

Gail Povar believes that these emotional responses and their associated barriers to good patient care can be reduced further by adhering to four management approaches: clarity, communication, caring, and closure.[3] *Clarity* involves a clear understanding by all parties regarding diagnosis, prognosis, therapeutic goals, and criteria used to judge when to withdraw treatment. Such plans should be reviewed and updated periodically as new information becomes available. *Communication* means that staff members and other caregivers should communicate important insights, be updated on changes, and be allowed to present concerns or reservations about the progress of treatment. *Caring* suggests that one recognize the emotional impediments to treatment removal and respond in a sensitive way. Such a response involves the patient, the family, and fellow caregivers who may be ambivalent about the removal of treatment. Finally, caregivers need *closure* by means of postmortem processing that reviews the caregiving process and allows for ethical reflection and enables the grieving process to occur.

These four management approaches will help people understand that there is no essential ethical difference between withholding and withdrawing treatment. The President's Commission points out that there is only one minor exception to this principle. When a caregiver offers a patient a treatment, additional expectations may arise regarding the obligation to continue treatment. Withdrawing treatment unilaterally is inappropriate because a significant aspect of the management plan is not shared with the patient and an implicit promise to the patient to continue treatment is abrogated. Therefore, caregivers should supply patients with information and involve them in a shared decision-making process so that the patient's best interests are served. Such an approach to information sharing implies that informed consent in these cases should be flexible and open to change consistent with new medical data.

Conclusion

Medicine deals not only with physical problems but with emotional considerations. Sound medical care takes emotional needs and opinions into account. Sound medical ethics requires a reasoned analysis as well, however. This chapter suggests that no ethical distinction exists between withdrawing and withholding treatment. Even though the two "feel" different, such feelings should not interfere with the appropriate ethical and medical care of the patient. Disagreements and confusion over removal of treatment in the clinical setting can be prevented by proper ethical analysis and certain practical approaches to patient care. Such approaches include ongoing comfort care and clear treatment goal setting, with the explicit understanding by all parties concerned that treatment can be removed if it is not benefiting the patient.

Notes

1. President's Commission for the Study of Ethical Problems in Medicine and Biomedical and Behavioral Research, *Deciding to Forgo Life-Sustaining Treatment* (Washington, D.C.: U.S. Government Printing Office, 1983), 77.
2. *Neurology* 39 (1989): 126.
3. Gail Povar, "Withdrawing and Withholding Therapy: Putting Ethics into Practice," *Journal of Clinical Ethics* 1 (spring 1990): 53.

Chapter 29 _____

Assessing Treatment Options

Over the past several years, there has been growing disaffection for paternalism in medical practice among physicians and patients alike. Underlying this disaffection has been an expanding societal awareness of and emphasis on individual rights and personal autonomy, as well as the emergence of a better-educated health care public. The result of these developments has been a recognition that decision making in health care is and must be a shared process between care provider and care receiver. Thus, patients and families are assuming more active roles in treatment decisions today than in the past. Within this changing environment, some physicians are becoming unsure of the requirements of their role with regard to such decisions.

Paralleling this development has been the rapid expansion of health care technologies. The scope of interventions available today includes the ability to visualize and measure physiological function in great detail; the capacity to gather, collate, and organize data to facilitate more efficient and comprehensive patient care; and the ability to substitute for lost function and circumvent the devastating effects of disease and disability. One predictable outcome of this trend has been a growing reliance on the ability of available technologies to overcome the otherwise natural restrictions that are part of the human condition. The danger of allowing the technological imperative—the belief that if we can do something we must, to prescribe use of these technologies—looms large in health care today.

When these tracks converge, two potentially troubling situations can arise. On the one hand, the physician may approach the patient—or in the event of the patient's incapacity, the family or other appropriate surrogate— and offer a variety of available therapies from which to choose. "This is what we can do. What do you want us to do for you or your loved one?" In such instances, patients and/or families are placed in the untenable position of having to make treatment decisions—a role for which they are neither prepared nor qualified. On the other hand, some physicians, fearful of the consequences of not giving adequate recognition to patient autonomy and self-determination, may find themselves ordering therapies that may not be medically indicated or appropriate but are provided because patients and/or families declare, "We want everything done." Neither approach is appropriate because neither recognizes the ethical limits associated with the goal of all decision making in health care: to contribute to the well-being of persons.

When a physician proposes some form of treatment to a patient, it should be with the hope that the regimen will provide benefit—that the patient will gain or at least maintain some ability to participate in and appreciate life and its attendant goods. In offering available treatment(s) to patients and/or families, then, the physician ought to give the best possible projections about hoped-for beneficial effects based on the physician's own considered judgment. That forecast certainly should include insight into the possible risks and/or burdens associated with the use of the therapy in question. Patients and families then weigh that information in light of their own values and goals and accept or refuse the proposed therapies.

Ought all available therapies be offered to patients and families? For example, should a patient who is in the terminal stages of cancer be offered cardiopulmonary resuscitation as a possibility in the event that cardiac or respiratory arrest occurs? Should renal dialysis be contemplated for the patient who has sustained profound and irreversible brain damage secondary to prolonged arrest? Should second or third liver transplants be made available to patients who have rejected the first liver and are statistically less apt to benefit from repeated transplant attempts? Often, lifesaving and life-sustaining therapies such as these are offered as possibilities to patients and families because the physician has failed to accept the responsibility to make some prior judgments about which of the available treatments are true options in a given case and which are not.

Principles

In making determinations about which available therapies or treatments are real options, physicians should be guided by two basic ethical principles. First, beneficence should lead the physician to consider as viable choices only therapies that offer some reasonable hope of providing benefit for the patient. Second, considerations of justice should prompt the care provider to recognize that in offering or providing therapies that are clearly nonbeneficial (e.g., dialysis for a person in persistent vegetative state), not only may the patient be harmed rather than helped but the broader society may be harmed because valuable and scarce resources may be wasted in the process.

Thus, some recognition of the limits that necessarily attend the practice of medicine, which ought to accompany the development and application of any medical technology and are a constitutive part of the human condition, must inform the assessment of treatment options. In entering into the caregiving relationship with patients and families, care providers should spend some time discussing the boundaries of what is possible, as well as what is beyond the realm of possibility in terms of treatment. Admittedly, these determinations are difficult to make. It is equally difficult to discuss the necessary limitations with patients and families, many of whom have come to believe that nothing is impossible in health care today. To neglect (worse, to deny) that such limits do exist, however, is to fail in the most basic obligation—namely, always to care.

When cure or meaningful amelioration of the effects of disease or disability is no longer reasonably possible, the physician or other care provider is obliged to recognize that the limits have been met. Therapies that provide little or no hope of benefit ought not be offered. Instead the physician should exercise his or her responsibility and prepare the patient and family for approaching death in these circumstances. Admitting and accepting the limitations of available therapies precludes the inappropriate physician response: "Here is what we can do . . . you choose what you want us to do for you or your loved one." In addition, when patients and families demand "we want everything done," it allows for the more fitting response: "We have done everything possible. There is nothing more we can do."

Conclusion

Two principle—beneficence and justice—ought to be operative when the physician makes a determination about which treatments are truly viable options for a particular patient. The former focuses appropriately on patient need as the primary concern. The latter directs attention to the needs of the broader community and requires that, in treating individual patients, the community's resources be used appropriately. Thus, when an available treatment or therapy can offer no reasonable hope of benefiting the patient, it should not be offered as a possibility. If physicians fail to exercise appropriate responsibility in this regard, society will make such determinations for them. When society makes these determinations, beneficence will not be the operative principle. Instead, economics will dictate treatment decisions.

Chapter 30

Discontinuing Life Support in Doubt

In Chattanooga, Tennessee, Gary Dockery—a policeman who was the victim of a gunshot wound to the head—started to speak after being almost totally nonresponsive for eight years. He regained limited speech, though he continues to be significantly paralyzed. Although descriptions of his original diagnosis seemed imprecise, his temporary recovery has been termed by family members as no less than a miracle.

In Moline, Michigan, Michael Martin existed in a debilitated state after being injured in a car/train collision. His injuries left him unable to walk, talk, or eat, and he required total care. He was conscious; he could nod, smile, and grip with his right hand. Despite his conscious state, the courts ruled him incompetent to make medical decisions. Although he never executed a written advance directive, his wife reported that he said that he would not have wanted to be kept alive in this type of compromised condition.

The Michigan Supreme Court has refused, however, to allow Mrs. Martin to authorize the removal of the feeding tube that is keeping her husband alive.

These two cases raise questions about the nature of surrogate decision making and the determination of a patient's best interests when there is doubt about the patient's prognosis and prior treatment desires. Additionally, in the latter case the ominous specter of the courts looms over the decision-making process. Is the judicial system, which offers legitimate protection for the weak, intervening inappropriately in a case like that of Mr. Martin?

Principles

Health care professionals employ two standard norms to determine when life-sustaining interventions may be forgone. First, treatments should not be utilized if they are ineffective in the sense that they offer no reasonable possibility for the patient to pursue goals or purposes in life. Second, treatments that inflict grave burdens in comparison with their benefits need not be used. A corollary derived from these two norms is that burdensome treatments that offer only a small statistical possibility of benefit (albeit significant benefit and even cure) need not be employed. Thus, one might not be obligated to take a treatment that offered a 1 percent chance of cure if it involved some burden because the treatment also has a 99 percent chance of failing. These norms provide the appropriate framework for evaluating surrogate decision making. The first norm, which focuses on quality of function, relies on more objective standards. The second norm and the correlative norm involve more subjective determinations that the patient or surrogate must calculate.

Health care workers generally respect the decisions of patients who speak for themselves with regard to their desire to receive or refuse treatment. Although these determinations involve a significant element of subjectivity, patients are usually best able to gauge benefit and burden in light of the probability of success. The situation becomes more convoluted, however, when patients lack the capacity to speak for themselves. Based on a desire to respect patient autonomy, proxies try to follow the patient's previously expressed desires. This standard for surrogate decision making is referred to as substituted judgment. Often, we know a patient's desire through a written directive (e.g., a living will or durable power of attorney for health care). More frequently, patients have verbally articulated wishes. Finally, we interpret the lifestyles of the patient to predict what the patient would have wanted. If this information is unavailable or inconclusive, proxies resort to a second standard—that of patient best interests. One tries to estimate what is likely to be in the patient's best interests by asking how the treatment will promote the patient's present and future welfare.

Unfortunately, a proxy decision likely will be less accurate than if the patient were to express his or her wishes directly. Written directives, although helpful, often may not take into account the complexities of the situation now at hand. Prior directives may not indicate the current interests of the incompetent patient. Moreover, proxies and physicians often fail to predict accurately a patient's wishes. Thus, one should move slowly and not instantly assign unlimited authority to proxy decision makers. Proxies may have other agendas or incorrectly project their own feelings onto the patient. Surrogate decisions should be scrutinized to ensure that they promote the wishes of the patient and the patient's best interests. At the very least, one should verify that a proxy's decision reflects an appropriate application of the norms governing the removal of life support.

Discussion

In Mr. Dockery's case, some confusion resulted because uncertainty existed about his exact condition. He was not in a classical coma, nor in a true persistent vegetative state, because he could at times respond to questions by blinking his eyes and uttering words. The patient apparently did not have any clear prior directives, so the family acted in what they thought were his best interests. Because there was hope that treatment would provide benefit, and treatment was not overtly harmful to him, the family decided it was in his best interests to continue to provide treatment. Yet family members also expressed concerns about providing aggressive care that offered a limited possibility of benefit. Had the treatment involved grave suffering, there might have been doubt about the wisdom of prolonged treatment. If that were the case, it would have been reasonable for the family to withdraw aggressive care even though in hindsight the intervention afforded him partial recovery. That is, a surrogate is not obligated to treat with the expectation that miracles will occur, especially when prolonged treatment inflicts a significant burden. The lack of statistical certitude in medicine necessarily leads to a certain ambiguity regarding the right choice to make. As a result, surrogates acting in good faith may make decisions that turn out to be inaccurate in retrospect.

In the case of Mr. Martin, the intervention of the Michigan court seems problematic. His wife indicated that her husband had previously expressed wishes indicating he would not want to be kept alive in such a debilitated condition. The court argued that he indicated his wishes regarding a vegetative state but not about his current condition. No directive, however, is able to take into account prospectively all possible situations. Holding a directive to that standard of evidence would be unreasonable. In addition, ethical analysis suggests that even without reference to previously expressed desires, one could make a compelling case that to continue treatment would not be in the best interests of the patient because of the burden and the lack of benefit of the treatment. Yet the court, citing a lack of an applicable patient directive, essentially rejected the substituted judgment standard and argued that continuing aggressive treatment is in the patient's best interests. This interpretation of "patient best interests" and the reluctance to discontinue treatment often originates from the emotional reluctance to remove artificial nutrition and hydration from a conscious patient, even though the removal of nutrition and hydration need not cause pain or suffering during the dying process if proper comfort care is given.

Supporters of the court's decision believe that it will deter inappropriate quality-of-life judgments for other people in debilitated states. Yet unlike some people who have been in debilitated conditions since birth and have not been able to express treatment preference, Mr. Martin had done that. Additionally, although one must work to prevent discrimination against severely handicapped individuals and outrageous quality-of-life judgments such as that in the infamous Indiana Baby Doe case, there may be times when proxies make a subjective determination that treatment has either become ineffective or is gravely burdensome in comparison with the benefit offered. One should not deny appropriate care for an individual because of a "slippery-slope" fear of inappropriate treatment for other persons in the future. One should deal with slippery-slope concerns separately. To use another man's life as a buffer to prevent future abuses is to use his life and his family as a means to an end.

Finally, in both of these situations, some people reason that the presumption to provide life support stems from the fact that if a judgment were in error and one were to discontinue treatment, there would be no going back. Yet moralists have never required the standard that people follow the safest course possible. Otherwise, it would be unethical to drive, cross the street, or engage in any type of "unnecessary" behavior that involves risk. Although one definitely should not forgo life support precipitously, neither should life be preserved at all costs.

Conclusion

When proxy decisions must be made, care must be taken not to act hastily. People who are conscious or semi-conscious yet incompetent must be given special protection because their vulnerability subjects them to possible discrimination. Sound application of the norms regarding the use of life support and the standards governing proxy consent should protect a patient's best interests. Although judicial interventions to protect patient rights in difficult cases may be warranted, the courts should "have their ethical act together." Court interventions that contradict ethical norms and common sense will serve only to compromise the care of patients in the long run. In particular, sentencing patients to medical limbo has already helped to generate calls for euthanasia. It may also cause families and patients to withhold or forgo truly beneficial care out of fear that once treatment is started, it may not be withdrawn even when it proves to be ineffective or gravely burdensome.

Chapter 31 _____

Religious Beliefs and Lifesaving Therapy

A forty-year-old St Louis woman and her fetus died after the woman refused a blood transfusion. As a member of the Jehovah's Witnesses, Bettye Joyce Beal believed that blood transfusions are prohibited by her religion. When she slipped and fell in her home, she began losing blood quickly. After she entered a hospital, doctors determined that the baby in her womb was not getting the blood and oxygen he needed. According to medical opinion offered in the press, mother and child might have survived if blood had been transfused at the proper time.

Ethics classes often consider the rights of Jehovah's Witnesses to refuse blood transfusions for themselves or their children as a problem in applying the principle of informed consent. This case provides some controversial aspects and an impetus to look more closely at the fundamental and related issues arising from the refusal to utilize a seemingly innocuous and success-ful life-prolonging therapy.

Principles

One of the most controversial ethical issues in the relationship between medicine and religion occurs when a Jehovah's Witness refuses a blood trans-fusion, even though death may occur as a direct result of this refusal. Clearly, the belief results in a confrontation between the Hippocratic oath and the individual's religious freedom. Physicians usually honor the patient's refusal on religious grounds to receive a blood transfusion because it is a legal prin-ciple of American society that people have a right to refuse medical treatment and because the ethics of medicine requires that therapy always be offered in accord with the spiritual or religious values of the person in question.

The belief that blood transfusions are contrary to biblical admonition is not shared by other Christian communities. True, certain passages of the Bible prohibit eating meat with blood still in it and drinking blood from animals offered in sacrifice to pagan gods.[1] Most biblical exegetes, how-ever, consider these prohibitions to be mere dietary laws that are no longer in effect or at most, laws that are directed to prohibiting idolatry. More important, the passages that prohibit eating or drinking blood say nothing about blood transfusions.

Richard Singelenberg reports that blood transfusions were not prohib-ited by the teaching authority of the Jehovah's Witnesses until 1945—well after the founding of that Church.[2] At first, Singelenberg maintains, "The Society hardly paid any attention to the new ruling," and "until the mid-forties the issues received only marginal attention in the Society's publica-tions." By the 1960s, however, the admonition concerning blood transfusions had consequence not only with regard to personal conscience; the Church also stated that accepting transfusions of blood would be followed by "dis-fellowshipping" (excommunication). Singelenberg attributes this prohibi-tion to social factors rather than the biblical interpretation. In sum, Singelenberg maintains that the prohibition of blood transfusions derives more from a desire to establish a practice that would separate Jehovah's Witnesses from the institutions of society (medicine being one of the promi-nent social institutions) than it does from a well-reasoned interpretation of pertinent scriptural passages.

Regardless of the history of the belief, refusing blood transfusions or ingestion of plasma or any other blood product clearly is a religious norm for a Jehovah's Witness who is seriously committed to the teaching of his or her Church. Is this belief a form of suicide? No: The intention of a Jehovah's Witness is to follow his or her faith. The fact that the person may die as a result of this choice is an indirect result of the choice to follow the faith teaching. For this reason, when Bettye Joyce Beal stated that she did not wish to have a blood transfusion even though her death would result, her wishes were honored.

Discussion

The Beal case is complicated immensely, however, by reason of the fact that Mrs. Beal's decision also affected the baby boy—Aviz by name—to whom she was about to give birth. Had she been given a transfusion before birth, the baby's chances of survival after a Caesarean section birth would have been better. After the birth, however, Roger Beal, the father of the child, told the medical staff that his "religion required that they not transfuse the child. That's what his mother would have wanted. I couldn't go against her." Should the wishes of Roger Beal have been honored even if Aviz, whose chances of survival by this time were slim, would die as a result of a low blood supply?

In considering the relationship between parents and children from the ethical perspective, two interrelated assumptions are paramount. First, the family unit must be fostered and protected because it is the fundamental element on which society and culture depend for strength and continuity. Second, parents should have care and custody of their children because experience shows that parents love their children and strive to help them become virtuous human beings. Like most ethical assumptions, however, this latter premise may yield to contrary evidence. For example, if parents are abusing their children and endangering their lives, society intervenes and removes the children from the parents' custody, at least for a time. The right of intervention on behalf of children illustrates another ethical assumption—namely, that parents do not "own" their children. Instead, parents are stewards or caretakers of their children, enablers who help their children grow in knowledge and virtue. Above all, life-and-death decisions concerning children are not to be made for the parents' benefit.

Ethical reasoning and legal precedent give priority to the expression of a person's religious faith. Because religious faith is the most personal, important, and profound act of conscience, its expression should be honored unless it is manifestly injurious to other people. Hence, as long as parents respect the well-being of their children, they have the ethical and legal right to rear and educate their children in the religion of the parents' choice.

The right to choose a religion for one's children, like many other parental rights, gradually wanes as the children mature and are able to make competent decisions for themselves. Here, of course, we encounter the crux of the matter: When are children able to make competent decisions for themselves? When do children become young adults? The laws of every country try to solve this question by stating that, for legal purposes, young people become adults at age 17, 18, or 21, depending on the right in question. (Strangely, in most U.S. states, young people may marry at an earlier age than they may buy alcoholic beverages.)

Such laws, however, express only a general norm; often a young person may be mature enough to make important decisions for himself or herself well before the legal age of maturity. In recognition of this fact, ethicists now suggest that teenage children be asked to give their "assent" to surgery or other serious medical treatments, even though the proxy consent of their parents or guardian will suffice for ethical and legal clearance for medical treatment.

Although judging the maturity of a teenager may be difficult, there is no quandary when infants are concerned. Clearly, they are unable to make mature judgments, and decisions concerning their well-being are the responsibility of their parents. If parents fail in their responsibility, the courts—acting in the name of society—are called upon to enter the decision-making process.

The habitual response of a court—the voice of society in regard to ethical behavior—is to grant permission for transfusions if the life of an infant is endangered. In fact, in emergencies this permission may be made by a medical team and reported later. The intent of the court is not to criticize the religious belief of the parents or the teaching of their church. Instead, the decision of the court is based on the fact that the children are not old enough to make a faith commitment of their own.

Conclusion

Aviz Beal was given a transfusion, but by the time he received it he was so compromised that he died shortly thereafter. Could the court have mandated that Mrs. Beal receive a transfusion before her death, when it might have done some good for the infant? Ethically speaking, a good case could have been made for transfusing Bettye Beal so that Aviz could live. Despite the abortion laws of the United States a mother has a moral responsibility to care for the child she carries in her womb. Practically speaking, however, it would be difficult to enforce a court order mandating transfusion for a pregnant woman.

Notes

1. Genesis 9:3–4; Acts 15:19–21; see also "How Can Blood Save Your Life?," (Watch Tower Society of New York, New York, 1990). See also Dridley, "Jehovah's Witnesses' Refusal of Blood." *Journal of Medical Ethics* 25 (1999): 469–72.
2. Richard Singelenberg, "The Blood Transfusion Taboo of Jehovah's Witnesses: Origin, Development, and Function of a Controversial Doctrine." *Social Science and Medicine* 4 (1990): 515–22.

Chapter 32 _____

Care for Patients in Persistent Vegetative States

The diagnosis, prognosis, and care of patients who are in a persistent vegetative state (PVS) has been an issue underlying much ethical and legal controversy. The decision of the Massachusetts Supreme Court in the Brophy case and the decision of the Missouri Supreme Court in the Cruzan case were diametrically opposed to each other. Yet both courts sought to base their decisions on the medical care suitable for patients in a PVS. Ethicists are also divided in regard to the proper care for patients in a PVS. Some ethicists maintain that all patients who are in a PVS should receive artificial hydration and nutrition because they will benefit from such treatment. Others maintain that such treatment is optional for patients in this condition because even though artificial hydration and nutrition circumvents a fatal pathology and extends life, it does not offer an overall benefit to the patient. This chapter presents the statement of the American

Academy of Neurology (AAN) regarding people in a PVS[1] and offers some ethical observations.

Principles

The AAN statement can be divided into three main sections: the medical description of a person in a PVS; the nature of artificial hydration and nutrition; and the use of artificial nutrition and hydration for a person in a PVS.

- *The medical description.* A patient who is in a PVS is permanently unconscious, with a functioning brain stem but a total loss of cerebral cortical functioning. Usually the person is able to breathe spontaneously but has no self-awareness; he or she is unable to perform voluntary actions and does not experience pain. The diagnosis of such a condition can be made with a high degree of medical certainty after a period of one to three months. Patients in a PVS may continue to survive for a prolonged period of time as long as artificial provision of nutrition and fluids is continued. Thus, because life support has been utilized, patients in this condition are not "terminally ill." The condition is permanent, however, because of the trauma and total loss of function in the cerebral cortex.
- *The nature of artificial hydration and nutrition.* Artificial provision of hydration and nutrition is a medical treatment rather than a nursing procedure; it is analogous to other forms of life-sustaining treatment, such as a respirator. When a patient is unconscious, a respirator and an artificial feeding device support or replace normal bodily functions that are compromised as a result of the patient's illness.
- *The use of artificial hydration and nutrition for patients in a PVS.* Good medical practice entails initiating hydration and nutrition when the patient's prognosis is uncertain but allows for termination if the patient's condition is hopeless (the family having been informed and consented to the withdrawal). Artificial hydration and nutrition may be discontinued in accordance with the principles and practices that govern the withholding and withdrawing of other forms of medical treatment: It should be based on a careful evaluation of the patient's diagnosis and prognosis, the prospective benefits and burdens of the treatment, and the stated preferences of the patient and family. When medical treatment fails to promote a patient's well-being, there is no longer any ethical obligation to provide

it. Medical treatment—including the provision of artificial nutrition and hydration—provides no hope for benefit to patients in a PVS once the diagnosis has been established to a high degree of medical certainty.

Discussion

Several points in the AAN statement are relevant from an ethical perspective. Because it is an ethical statement by physicians concerning an important and difficult issue in medical care, it is worthy of note. For too long judges, lawyers, theologians, and ethicists have analyzed contentious issues in medicine, and many scientists and physicians have acted as though their profession were "value free." Without denying the contribution of ethics and law to the solution of issues arising from medical care, the voice of medicine must be heard as well if a well-balanced and clinical view of these human problems is to develop. Physicians' groups should apply themselves to other ethical issues associated with medicine, such as access to health care.

The statement that artificial hydration and nutrition is a medical treatment similar to the use of a respirator is welcome because it offers a model for decision making that most people can understand. The great contribution of the AAN statement, however, is the simple syllogism: Medical treatment attempts to promote the well-being of the patient. Artificial hydration and nutrition does not promote the well-being of a person in a PVS. Therefore, artificial hydration and nutrition may be withheld from a patient who is in a PVS.

The statement contains no hint of approval of active or passive euthanasia. The reason for withdrawing treatment from a patient who is permanently unconscious is not based on a quality-of-life argument. Treatment is withdrawn by analyzing the quality of the means insofar as the condition of the patient is concerned. When artificial hydration and nutrition are withdrawn, the family and physicians do not intend death and do not *cause* death. Death is caused by the underlying pathology: the inability to chew and swallow. The intention of the family and physician is to avoid doing something that would be useless or would impose an excessive burden on the patient.

Grasping the distinction between avoiding harm to the patient (a good act) and causing the patient's death (an evil act) is difficult for many people when artificial hydration and nutrition are in question. The main reason for this difficulty seems to be that death occurs inevitably when the artificial hydration and nutrition are removed, no matter what the motive underlying the removal might be. Human actions receive their designation as good or evil from the effect of the action and the intention of the person performing or withholding the action, however, not from the accidental effects of the action. Hence, if the proximate motive for removing hydration and nutrition is to avoid harming the patient, the ensuing death—because it is not intended—is extraneous to the moral evaluation of the act. One way to help people make a good ethical decision about removing life support is to ask, "Would you remove this life support even if it would not result in the patient's death?"

Conclusion

For many reasons, the AAN statement is welcome and enlightening. Yet the statement alone will not lead to consensus. We need more discussion and common understanding of issues such as quality of life, the nature of a moral act, what constitutes the well-being of a patient, and causing death as distinguished from allowing death to occur naturally when there is no moral imperative to prolong life.

Note

1. Executive Board, American Academy of Neurology. "Position of the American Academy of Neurology on Certain Aspects of the Care and Management of the Persistent Vegetative State Patient," *Neurology* 39 (January 1989): 125–27.

Chapter 33 _____

Unfinished Business in the Cruzan Case

In November 1990 Charles Teel, judge of the circuit court of Jasper County in the state of Missouri, once again heard the petition of Joe and Joyce Cruzan to remove life support from their daughter Nancy Beth, who had been seriously injured in an automobile accident in 1983. Declaring that there was "clear and convincing" evidence of her wishes not to exist in a persistent vegetative state, on December 14, 1990, Judge Teel declared that artificial hydration and nutrition could be withdrawn from Nancy Beth. Nancy Beth Cruzan died of natural causes on December 26, 1990.

William Webster, the attorney general of Missouri, did not appeal this second decision of Judge Teel. He did appeal Judge Teel's first decision, however; as a result, the case went to the Missouri Supreme Court and eventually to the U.S. Supreme Court. The U.S. Supreme Court agreed that the Missouri Supreme Court had the right to require "clear and convincing evidence" before allowing the removal of life support from unconscious people. The U.S. Supreme Court did not review the ethical reasoning of the Missouri Supreme Court, however. It is time to review and renounce that reasoning, else other families will suffer the same injustice that befell the Cruzans.

Clearly, court decisions are based on legal precedent more than on ethical reasoning. Some reliance on ethical reasoning is required, however, to formulate equitable court decisions. As the Missouri Supreme Court stated in the Cruzan case, "We remain true to our role only if our decision is firmly founded on legal principle and reasoned analysis." Reasoned analysis is another term for ethical reasoning. What was the ethical reasoning underlying the Missouri Supreme Court decision in the Cruzan case?

Three Assumptions

Three assumptions underlie the efforts of the Missouri Supreme Court at ethical reasoning. All three assumptions seem deficient in light of ethical norms for removing life support from people who suffer from a fatal pathology. First, the court assumes that allowing a person to die because therapy is ineffective is the same as killing the person: "This is not a case in which we are asked to let someone die. . . . This is a case in which we are asked to allow the medical profession to make Nancy die by starvation and dehydration." Making someone die or causing the death of another person means that the agent of the action intends the death of the other person and, by placing or omitting actions, brings about death. When a person will not benefit from medical care, however, the intention of people removing treatment is not to bring about death but to admit that the illness or pathology threatening death cannot be treated in a manner that is beneficial for the patient. When life support is removed from a patient because it is not beneficial, we are simply admitting the limits of human ingenuity and medical science. Many times people express such intentions when support is removed from loved ones, uttering such phrases as, "We cannot help Mom anymore," or, "Dad wouldn't want to live in this condition."

Although the distinction between intending death and admitting human limitations is fine, it is realistic. Good ethical distinctions are as fine as silk and as strong as steel. In the case of persons in a persistent vegetative state (PVS) or in other conditions in which therapy is ineffective or would impose a grave burden, removing life support does not cause death. Instead, removing life support allows death to occur as the result of a natural pathology that is not beneficial to resist. There is no moral imperative to prevent people from dying if they are in a PVS or suffer from other severely debilitating conditions from which they will not recover. Moreover, the Missouri court's statement that Nancy Beth Cruzan would die of starvation and dehydration if life support were removed is inaccurate, as well as inflammatory. This language brings to mind a vision of a conscious and healthy person dying an excruciating death because she is deprived of beneficial care. Reference to "starvation and dehydration" of patients in a PVS has little relation to reality. People in a PVS die because of injury to their cerebral cortex. Just as they can no longer chew or swallow, they do not feel pain.[1]

The second assumption underlying the decision of the Missouri Supreme Court in the Cruzan case is that persons suffering from fatal pathologies must be kept alive as long as possible. The court expresses this assumption by consistently referring to the fact that Nancy "is not terminally ill"; for this reason, it would not allow the removal of life support. Others repeated this error by stating, "Nancy is not dying." Both statements imply, however, that Nancy's fatal pathology would be assessed ethically only after life support has been utilized. To be "terminally ill" in the mind of the Missouri Supreme Court means that a person will die even if life support has been applied. Under this assumption respirators, dialysis, and especially artificial hydration and nutrition should not be removed unless they fail to prolong life.

In assessing whether to use or continue life support, however, the essential issue is not whether life can be prolonged but whether life should be prolonged. Will the person benefit if life is prolonged? In ethical reasoning, the questions "Will the life support impose a grave burden?" and "Will the life support be effective?" are asked before life support is utilized. As the Illinois Supreme Court stated of terminal illness, "This assessment of imminence renders the definition of a terminal illness circular and meaningless and makes it impossible for compassionate care for people unable to benefit from therapy. Imminence must be judged as if the death-delaying procedures were absent."[2] One hopes that this insight with regard to "terminal illness," which is more in accord with ethical reasoning, will become accepted across the country. If it were, much of the misunderstanding and contention that surrounds the removal of life support could be obviated.

The third assumption underlying the Missouri court's decision was that "the state's interest is not in the quality of life. The state's interest is an unqualified interest in life." *If quality of life* implies impaired function as a result of serious pathology, and if the state has no interest in quality of life, then every means possible must be utilized to prolong the life of every person suffering from any impaired function whatsoever. How severely impaired the person might be would not matter, as long as the person could be kept alive. According to this thinking, we should consider kidney transplants for people in a PVS who have end-stage renal disease and heart transplants for people in a PVS who have chronic cardiomyopathy. Although these conclusions are ludicrous, they are in accord with the court's reasoning. All other state courts that have rendered decisions in PVS cases have admitted a reasonable limit to state interest in the face of seriously impaired function. As Judge Blackmar pointed out in his dissent to the majority opinion in the Cruzan case, if Missouri has an unqualified interest in preserving life, how can we explain the existence of capital punishment and the living will law in Missouri?

Conclusion

As we insist that the ethical reasoning of the Missouri Supreme Court be revised, let us ask another question: Is the court the place to decide questions about prolonging life for persons who are severely debilitated as the result of fatal pathologies? Questions of this nature have been settled in the family forum for years. Does the court do a better job than the family? The family forum is public; not only family members but physicians, nurses, clergy, and others are involved in the ultimate decision. Moreover, the family forum has a more humane and compassionate motivation than the legal forum. Rather than being mainly concerned with state interest and legal precedent, the family forum is concerned with doing what is best for the patient.

Notes

1. Executive Board, American Academy of Neurology. "Position of the American Academy of Neurology on Certain Aspects of the

Care and Management of the Persistent Vegetative State Patient,"
Neurology 39 (January 1989): 125–27.
2. Supreme Court of Illinois, *In re Estate of Sidney Greenspan* 146, Ill,
D.E.C. 860, 558 NE 2nd, 1194, July 9, 1990.

Chapter 34

"Only God Can Heal My Daughter"

While treating twelve-year-old Pamela Hamilton for a broken leg, Pamela's
physician discovered a cancerous tumor, which was diagnosed as Ewing's
sarcoma. Larry Hamilton—Pamela's father and pastor at the Church of
God of the Union Assembly in La Follette, Tennessee—and her mother,
Deborah, refused treatment of Pamela's cancer because taking medicine is
against their religion. "Only God can heal my daughter," declared her
father; "She has the faith to recover; it will be God's will if she does not."
Having been notified of Pamela's condition, the Tennessee Department of
Social Service petitioned the courts for custody of Pamela on the grounds
that her life was endangered because of her parents' religious beliefs. By the
time the courts of Tennessee granted the transfer of custody, two months
had elapsed. The attending physician stated that she had only a 50 percent
chance of survival because of the "red hot and angry tumor which now has
spread through her thigh and up to the hip joint." Even though her life was
endangered, Pamela agreed with her parents' decision and declared, "I do
not want radiation and chemotherapy because I do not want my hair to fall
out or to be sick."

In fact Pamela died within one year after chemotherapy began. The
tumor was too far advanced for successful therapy.

Principles

In considering the relationship between parents and children from
the Judeo-Christian ethical perspective, two interrelated assumptions are

paramount. First, the family unit must be fostered and protected because it is the fundamental element on which society and culture depend for strength and continuity. Second, parents should have care and custody of their children because experience shows that parents love their children and strive to help them become virtuous human beings. Like most ethical assumptions, this latter premise may yield to contrary evidence. If parents are abusing their children and endangering their lives, society intervenes and removes the children from the parents' custody, at least for a time. The right of intervention on behalf of children illustrates another ethical assumption—namely, that parents do not "own" their children. Parents are stewards or caretakers of their children, enablers who help their children grow in knowledge and virtue. Above all, life-and-death decisions concerning children are not to be made for the parents' benefit.

Ethical reasoning and legal precedent give priority to the expression of a person's religious faith. Because religious faith is the most personal, important, and profound act of conscience, its expression should not be limited unless it is manifestly injurious to other people. Hence, as long as parents respect the well-being of their children, they have the ethical and legal right to rear and educate their children in the religion of the parents' choice. The right to choose a religion for children, like many other parental rights, gradually wanes as children mature and are able to make competent decisions for themselves.

Here, of course, we encounter the crux of the matter: When are children able to make competent decisions for themselves? When do children become young adults? The laws of every country try to solve this question by stating that, for legal purposes, young people become adults at age 17, 18, or 21, depending on the right in question. (Strangely, in most U.S. states, young people may marry at an earlier age than they may buy alcoholic beverages.) These laws, however, express only a general norm; often a young person may be mature enough to make important decisions for himself or herself well before the legal age of maturity. In recognition of this fact, ethicists now suggest that capable children be asked to give their "assent" to surgery or other serious medical treatments, even though the proxy consent of their parents or guardian will suffice for ethical and legal clearance for medical treatment.

Discussion

Cases resembling that of Pamela Hamilton are not unusual. Courts frequently appoint guardians for children whose parents are Jehovah's

Witnesses who believe that the Bible prohibits blood transfusions even when death would occur without them. The ethical basis for court action is the assumption that the child's life should not be endangered by the parent's religious beliefs. Even if the child agrees with the parents' beliefs, the ethical and legal thinking in most of these cases is that the child cannot make a competent decision and that, because life is such as important gift, he or she would choose life if a competent and free decision were possible.

Pamela's situation was different from the usual transfer-of-custody case for religious reasons. First, she agreed with her parents' decision that she should not receive medicine for treatment of cancer. On the face of it, the parents' statement that "God will cure." is unreasonable. Although religious people attribute omnipotence to God and, in that sense, believe that God does cure, they usually do not deny that human beings have a cooperative role to fulfill in effecting a cure. That human beings will one day die is assured, but they have a right and a duty to use positive means such as medicine and surgery to prolong their lives as long as living enables them to pursue the goal of life. Yet even if the belief of Pamela and her parents seems unreasonable, their religious belief should be honored unless it manifestly harms other people.

This analysis brings us to the second issue that makes Pamela's case different: There was a threat that she would die within a year even if chemotherapy and radiation were used. The fact that she might survive does not obviate the need for the court to ask, at the time of the original discussion, What if we take her from her family, give her extensive chemotherapy, and she dies anyway?

In most states, if Pamela were more than eighteen years old and stated that because of her religious beliefs she did not wish to receive medical treatment for her tumor, people might try to persuade her to change her mind, but ultimately they would be legally and ethically bound to respect her decision. The question that bothers us is this: Even though she is only twelve years old, did the court make an effort to determine her maturity? No doubt Pamela's faith is strong, but is it based on her parents' influence or her own free convictions? Furthermore, did the court consider the gravity of her condition before making its decision?

Conclusion

Given the choice, most people will choose life over death, and legal precedent must be based on what happens most of the time. Legal precedent alone, however, does not guarantee an ethical solution. An ethical solution requires that legal precedent be interpreted in light of the pertinent facts of the case and the ethical assumptions on which the precedent is based. Pamela's case reminds us that religious and family rights are very important and that the courts must consider particular facts and assumptions as well as precedent to make ethical decisions.

Chapter 35

It's Time to Resolve the "Futility Debate"

Discussions about doing or not doing futile things have been part of medicine since its beginnings. Only recently, however, have such deliberations been elevated to the status of a "debate." Thus, in cases such as those involving Helga Wanglie and Baby K, physicians, ethicist, and the courts have argued the merits of providing versus withholding or withdrawing life-sustaining interventions even when the condition of the patient is irremediable. Although one can learn a great deal from examining cases such as these, conferring "debate" status on the discussions gives the impression that doing what is useless may be appropriate at times. In fact, in the Wanglie and Baby K cases, the courts mandated that life-sustaining interventions be continued even though the interventions offered no hope of changing the condition of the patient in question.

Debating futility and its relation to medical practice is a misguided effort that is not fitting for people who are concerned about human well-being. Medicine has an intrinsic *telos* or goal, and the aimless use of medical resources transgresses that goal. Moreover, futile use of life-sustaining interventions violates the good and well-being of individual persons as well as the community of persons. An examination of why this debate rages— more precisely, why futile treatments are pursued—as well as the consequences of futile treatments bears this out.

Doing and Debating What Is Futile

The futility debate results first from a failure to appreciate the proper goals or ends of medicine. As a profession, medicine exists to promote the health—the integrated functioning—of persons. Physicians assess and use medical resources toward this end. Because appropriate use of these resources is determined best by persons who are knowledgeable about things medical, physicians' medical judgments should not be displaced by the uninformed though well-meaning desires of persons who are not physicians. In other words, some decisions about the use of medical resources should be made solely by physicians. Among these decisions are judgments about what proposed medical interventions can and cannot do in light of a patient's diagnosis and condition.

Second, the futility debate results in large part from an inadequate understanding of personal autonomy and individual rights. Thus, in the case of Helga Wanglie, a statement made by Mrs. Wanglie to her husband before she became ill was construed by the court as binding on medical personnel even though her condition had deteriorated to the point that any further intervention could only sustain her in a persistent vegetative state. Although her physiological life could be prolonged, there was no possibility of integrated function; thus, no medical intervention could achieve its intended goal. Adequate regard for an individual's autonomy and rights does not require that physicians act beyond that which is reasonable or consistent with good medicine.

Third, the tendency among some physicians to abdicate their legitimate authority and allow patients and/or families to make decisions that they are not equipped to make contributes to the use of futile interventions. Rather than relying on appropriate medical criteria to limit the range of available interventions to those that offer some reasonable hope of promoting integrated function, some physicians simply ask patients and/or families, "What do you want me to do?" This approach often gives the false impression that there is reason for hope even in situations in which there is none. In such circumstances, distressed patients and/or families frequently respond, "Do everything!" Unfortunately, in many situations doing "everything" serves only to prolong dying—and, at times, to increase suffering.

Fourth, overestimation of the legal system's ability to adjudicate difficult cases involving the use or non-use of life-sustaining interventions contributes significantly to the use of futile interventions. Although the courts may have some limited role in making treatment-related decisions, they should never be used as a means of circumventing appropriate medical authority. That is precisely what happened in the Wanglie case, in which the court decreed that Mrs. Wanglie's stated preferences should be followed regardless of medical data indicating the futility of doing so.

Finally, the debate about futility seems to be a symptom of a pervasive societal fascination with matters of dying. On the one hand, proposals continue to be made to legalize physician-assisted suicide to enable patients to escape the protracted dying that many persons fear. On the other hand, many people are arguing that prolonging the dying process should be an option that persons may choose in light of their own perspectives and values.

Consequences of Doing Medically Futile Things

Regardless of the reasons, when futile interventions are provided, significant consequences ensue not only for patients but for families, health care professionals, and society. Consider the effects on patients and families. Dying persons often suffer needlessly because of the demands for continued interventions made by themselves or ill-informed loved ones. As a result, death often occurs incrementally, an organ or organ system at a time. In such circumstances, experiencing dying as a personal reality is not possible. There is little ability to allow for "a good death" in these cases. In addition, providing future interventions at the end of life often requires that care be rendered in a highly technological environment that may not welcome the caring, concerned presence of loved ones. Dying under such circumstances can be a very lonely, isolating experience for patients and families. Moreover, when unreasonable efforts to sustain life are made, appropriate concern seldom is given to preparing patients or their families for death. Little if any attention is paid to strengthening relationships and "putting affairs in order" or to spending quality time with loved ones. As a result, when death does occur, there is little left but anguish and regret. When physicians acquiesce to the demands of patients, families, or the courts and provide interventions that they deem futile, families often gain a renewed sense of hope in situations in which continued hope is inappropriate. There are times in the course of serious illness when hope must give way to acceptance and resignation so necessary preparations can be made. In hopeless situations, families need assistance in coming to grips with the reality of loss so that they can grieve appropriately and, after a time, get on with their lives.

Health care professionals are not immune to the ill effects of the futility trap. Medicine is an inherently goal-oriented profession. When physicians and other health professionals are compelled to do useless, often harmful things to patients, many feel ethically compromised. Moreover, recognizing that they are dispensing very valuable resources in a useless endeavor is a demoralizing realization. This awareness can be particularly painful for physicians given the increasing awareness about the cost of health care and concerns about equitable access to basic services. Finally, when physicians, nurses, and others do futile things, for whatever reason, they often feel more like technicians than true professionals. The problem is that there is no mandate that technicians be motivated by altruism or interest in the well-being of those they serve. The danger, of course, is that professions that are threatened today on many fronts will be further compromised and less likely to survive intact in the future.

Society is affected adversely by allowing the futility debate to continue unchecked. When legitimate professional authority is subjugated to the idiosyncratic preferences of autonomous individuals, society loses an effective voice for reason in the wise use of society's resources. When society's health care resources are expended in futile and useless interventions on behalf of individuals, the community as a whole pays the price. One result is that vulnerable persons—those in need of health care services who have neither the resources nor the voice to access the system—are made even more vulnerable. Finally, the propensity to do futile things in medicine, for whatever reason, reinforces the pervasive societal aversion to deal appropriately with human dying and contributes to proposals to kill rather than compassionately care for those at life's end.

Conclusion

Several factors have contributed to a concision of roles and responsibilities with regard to decisions about the appropriate use of medical resources. Among these factors are our fascination with individual rights and a desire to "level the playing field" in matters of decision making and our fascination with technology coupled with an unwillingness to accept the limits of our mortality. One result of this growing confusion has been the conviction that the appropriateness of doing futile things in medicine merits continued debate. It is time, however, to resolve the futility debate by realizing that failure to do so is harmful for the whole community of persons.

Chapter 36 _____

Court Decisions on Futile Therapy

When do physicians and hospitals have the right to deny health care that proxies for incapacitated patients desire but health care professionals consider to be futile? A Massachusetts court recently issued a ruling in this regard. Catherine Gilgunn became comatose and suffered irreversible neurological damage.[1] Mrs. Gilgunn's daughter, Joan Gilgunn, maintained that her mother had always wanted "everything done" to prolong her life even if she became mentally incompetent. Even in the face of this knowledge, the attending physician—after consulting the hospital's ethics committee—wrote a "do not resuscitate" (DNR) order for Mrs. Gilgunn. The ethics committee's decision was based on the opinion that resuscitation would not benefit Mrs. Gilgunn and was therefore futile.

Shortly after the DNR order was written, Mrs. Gilgunn died. Her daughter sued the hospital and the doctor, maintaining that refusal to provide care requested by patients or their families constituted malpractice, regardless of the medical condition of the patient. The jury returned an innovative verdict. The judge asked them to consider whether Mrs. Gilgunn, if she had been able to speak for herself, would have chosen to be resuscitated. The jury responded in the affirmative. The judge then asked the jury whether the attempts to resuscitate Mrs. Gilgunn would have been futile, and the jury again answered in the affirmative. Based on this analysis, the jury acquitted the attending physician and the hospital.

Principles

Informed consent, whether offered by patients or their proxies, is based on the notion that medical care should respect the dignity of the patient. Respecting the dignity of patients requires that patients or their proxies be allowed to make autonomous decisions about medical care. Hence, an essential element of informed consent is allowing the patient or proxy to select or reject therapy. Thus, preserving autonomy through informed consent becomes a predominant interest insofar as medical therapy is concerned.

With this background in mind, courts in the United States in several well-publicized cases have required physicians and hospitals to continue treatment regardless of the condition of the patient if treatment is requested by the patient's proxy. In the Baby K and Wanglie cases, for example, courts in Minnesota and Virginia declared that life-prolonging therapy should be continued even though the health care professionals judged such care to be futile. In other prominent cases, such as the Cruzan case, the courts decided that life-prolonging therapy must be continued unless there was clear and convincing evidence that the patient would want it discontinued. Thus, the Cruzan family—who were the proxies for Nancy Beth—were not allowed to speak on her behalf because they did not have legal documents expressing her wishes. In sum, legal decisions in the United States have been heavily weighted in favor of continuing therapy if it is requested by patient or proxy even if the health care professionals believe the therapy in question to be futile.

Physicians and hospital administrators often object to providing therapy they deem futile even if this therapy is requested. The tendency to declare some therapy *futile* is relatively recent. Previously, therapy would be withheld if it was considered ineffective insofar as reversing an imminently fatal pathology was concerned. The term *futile* was not used to justify withholding or withdrawing therapy. Accurately defining *futile therapy* has been a problem. Some commentators maintain the need to distinguish between futile *care* and futile *therapy*. Care is never futile, they maintain, but therapy may be deemed futile if it does not achieve the purpose for which it is utilized. The concept of futile therapy introduces discussion about the overall purpose of medicine. Does therapy fulfill the purpose of medicine if it merely maintains physiological function but has no hope of restoring cognitive-affective function? Some physicians and ethicists maintain that unilateral decisions may be made to withdraw or withhold life-sustaining therapy if the therapy is judged to be futile by the health care professional responsible for the patient. Those who hold this opinion do not consider informed consent—that is, the ability to choose or reject therapy—an absolute right. Those who reject the concept of futile therapy are stating, at least implicitly, that the goal of medicine is to prolong the life of patients as long as possible, no matter how debilitated the function of the patient.

Discussion

Who has the right to decide that a particular form of medical therapy is futile? Basically, this decision is the responsibility of the attending physician, although important decisions of this nature should be made in consultation with others. First and foremost, the persons who speak for incapacitated patients should be involved in the decision. If a legal document such as a durable power of attorney is applicable, the designated agent should be consulted. If a legal document has not been signed, a family member usually has the moral right to speak for the incapacitated person. Experience demonstrates that physicians and proxies can often be assisted in their deliberations by an ethical consultant, a pastoral care person, or by members of an ethics committee. For best results, such consultants should be involved before an impasse is reached between the physician and the family. Agreement concerning futile therapy is usually possible. Only as a last resort should a disagreement over futile therapy be taken to court.

The Gilgunn case is worthy of note because cases of this nature do not occur frequently. Usually, physicians are willing to follow the wishes of a proxy in cases of futile therapy, thinking that the issue may resolve itself through the impending death of the patient. Other cases never reach a courtroom because the legal resolution of an ethical issue is a cumbersome and usually unsatisfying process. Cases involving futile care that do reach a court are concerned with persons who will never regain cognitive-affective function. For these persons, it seems fair to say that there is such a thing as futile therapy.

The lawyers alleging malpractice in the Gilgunn case implied that physicians are simply the servants of the patients; physicians must do whatever the patient or proxy requests. Moreover, they alleged that the reason resuscitation was withheld was because Mrs. Gilgunn was old and unimportant. The lawyer for the family stated, "Who is going to miss Mrs. Gilgunn? She was old and not very productive and had very little family. When it comes to decisions like this, we can't presume to take away a person's right to make treatment decisions merely to get people out of hospitals."

The thoughts expressed by the lawyers for the family underline the need to ensure that decisions concerning futile care are made for the right reasons. Economic factors alone do not constitute sufficient reason for declaring a therapy to be futile. True, a therapy may be declared unavailable in a particular case because it is too expensive. That judgment, however, is not the same as determining that a therapy is futile. Life-prolonging health care must not be withheld from elderly people simply because they are old or nonproductive. The only appropriate reason for withdrawing or withholding care when futile therapy is in question is because it will not benefit the patient. Benefit results when therapy enables a person to pursue the goods of life. Even debilitated and nonproductive patients may pursue the goods of life and thus should be given life-prolonging therapy if there is some hope that it will benefit them. Usually, if therapy is requested by a patient or proxy, there is an assumption that such therapy will help the patient pursue the goods of life. When one has lost the capacity to pursue the goods of life—when the power to think, love, and relate to others will never be restored—therapy that will prolong physiological function alone becomes futile therapy. If the patient in question has not lost cognitive-affective function permanently, deciding that therapy is futile is much more difficult.

Conclusion

Will the decision of the court in Massachusetts change the thinking of courts in other states with regard to judgments about futile care? Hardly! The decision in question was an answer to a malpractice charge. It did not concern a constitutional right, nor did it probe other foundational issues. By inference and implication, however, the decision of the jury in Massachusetts might have some effect with regard to ethical deliberations. The decision implies that physicians are on safe ground ethically if they decide that some forms of therapy are futile, even if the proxy requests them for a patient. Clearly, this judgment is a departure from the practice of the past.

Note

1. Gina Kolata, "Court Ruling Limits Rights of Patients," *New York Times,* June 5, 1995.

Chapter 37 _____

The Wanglie Case: Demands for Futile Therapy

A few years ago, a Minnesota judge granted guardianship to Helga Wanglie's husband and directed physicians to comply with Mr. Wanglie's demands for continued life-sustaining care for his wife. Three days later, Mrs. Wanglie died of sepsis while still on full life support in an intensive care unit. In rendering its decision, the court focused primary attention on the locus of decision making. As a result, the significance of the content of the demands being made by Mrs. Wanglie's family were minimized. The fact that the interventions in question had been judged medically futile by the physicians caring for Mrs. Wanglie apparently was not a central concern in the court's decision.

The ruling in the Wanglie case reflects a growing sentiment that medical decisions about the good of the patient should be reached by consideration of subjective data alone—that is, the personal values of the patient or family—with little or no reference to any objective information or input provided by the physician. From this perspective, doing what is right and good for persons involves little more than responding to their expressed wants and desires. Thus, the court's decision in the Wanglie case questions the body of knowledge at the heart of medicine. This knowledge does provide objective data for making determinations about human good and how to promote it. The pervasiveness of the attitude reflected in the finding of the court threatens to enervate the profession of medicine and undermine its basic commitment to human good and well-being.

Mrs. Wanglie's ordeal began when she fractured her hip. Shortly after the surgical repair of the fracture, she began a downhill course that eventually left her persistently vegetative secondary to severe hypoxic encephalopathy. Her physical condition was such that continued physiological life required full technical support and ongoing intensive care. Although physicians repeatedly informed the family of Mrs. Wanglie's poor prognosis and made it clear that continued medical intervention would do nothing to reverse her neurological status or improve her overall condition, her husband, daughter, and son insisted that full support be continued. Mr. Wanglie argued that the family's position reflected his wife's earlier statement that "if anything happened to her so that she could not take care of herself, she did not want anything done to shorten or prematurely take her life."

In ordering physicians to carry out Mr. Wanglie's demands for continued life-sustaining interventions, the court obviated consideration of the central issue: the questionable appropriateness of allowing and encouraging patients or their surrogates to demand and receive interventions that are judged to be medically futile. To discuss the significance of this case, we must explore the meaning of futility as it relates to medical care and examine the implications of the court's decision for the future of medical practice.

Futility and the Practice of Medicine

"Futile" describes something that is frivolous, trivial, without meaning, or of no consequence. Applied to specific human activity, futility delineates actions that offer no reasonable possibility of accomplishing the goals for which they are performed. In the context of medical practice, *futility* is used to describe interventions that do not offer a reasonable hope of contributing to the integrated functioning of the person. Medical interventions of the kind used for Mrs. Wanglie (e.g., mechanical ventilator, feeding tube, vasopressor drugs) are not prescribed by the physician solely to address physiological problems. In seeking the good of the person, the physician renders medical care in the hope of alleviating a physiological problem *in order to promote the integrated functioning of the whole person* (i.e., integration of the physiological, psychological, social, and creative dimensions)—thus allowing the person some capacity to pursue life's goals and objectives.

Although an antibiotic may be successful in treating pneumonia, it would be a futile intervention for a person whose overall condition does not allow for integrated functioning—for example, when the person is in a persistent vegetative state (PVS). In a PVS irreversible loss of function of the cerebral cortex precludes integration of the psychological, social, and creative dimensions of the person. Although the physiological level of function of a person in a PVS can be affected, the person herself cannot pursue human objectives because of the underlying physical condition. On the other hand, although an antibiotic used to treat pneumonia in a person in the terminal stage of cancer cannot reverse the course of the cancer, it may afford the person the opportunity to strive for his or her objectives in life in a limited way. In the latter case, the conclusion that the intervention is not futile and can be offered to the patient depends on the overall condition of the person and his or her capacity for some degree of integrated function even in the presence of terminal disease. In the latter example, although the physician makes the determination that the proposed therapy may offer a reasonable hope of benefit for the patient, it is then up to the patient or proxy to accept or refuse the therapy based on his or her own assessment of potential benefit and associated burden.

Determinations of medical futility are based on clinical data (the findings of physical examination, laboratory reports, x-ray results, etc.) as well as the experience of the clinician in applying similar therapies in similar cases. Thus, the judgment that a given therapy is medically futile is a description of the objective quality of the therapy relative to a given patient in light of the patient's medical condition. For this reason, the determination that a therapy or medical intervention is medically futile rests with the physician alone. Once such a conclusion has been reached, the physician should not be compelled to offer or provide the intervention.

This conclusion is challenged by persons who argue that physicians and patients may value different outcomes in the medical encounter. Although the physician may conclude that continued efforts to preserve the physiological function of a person in an irreversible coma are not justified, some patients and families may believe otherwise. Thus, in the case of Mrs. Wanglie, the family insisted that continued physiological function was what they wanted even if maintained function could not serve Mrs. Wanglie's overall well-being. The fact that a patient or family wants an outcome, however, does not legitimate the pursuit of that outcome—particularly when such pursuit requires ongoing medical care provided by and within a community of persons and the use of medical resources.

Conclusion

The determination that an available therapy is medically futile is a professional judgment that is based on verifiable medical data about the potential of a given intervention to affect the overall, integral well-being of the patient. This concern for and commitment to the good of the patient is at the heart of the medical profession. Although individual physicians may have subjective feelings about particular patient outcomes (e.g., that life in a PVS is "not worth living"), there is no evidence to suggest that determinations of medical futility, as in the Wanglie case, are shaped by the personal values of physicians. Neither should we conclude that reliance on physician judgment in determining medical futility threatens to undermine the rights and values of the patient or family in the caregiving relationship. Rather, supporting the physician in doing what she or he is educated to do in the context of the care-giving relationship ensures that patient good and well-being will continue to be at the heart of medical practice. The physician's role is to make reasoned decisions that are based on sound medical knowledge, to seek consultation to verify findings, and to recommend only interventions that offer some reasonable hope of benefit. Compelling physicians to offer and provide therapies that, in their best medical judgment, are not conducive to the overall good of the patient risks changing the nature and focus of the caregiving relationship—as well as the nature of the medical profession itself.

Chapter 38

Baby K: It's Time to Take a Stand

Baby K is a sixteen-month-old anencephalic girl who has been kept alive by means of aggressive life support. The child lives in a nursing home and has recurrent bouts of respiratory distress requiring emergency room treatment at the regional medical center in Falls Church, Virginia. The hospital physicians believe that the care is futile and should not be continued. The mother, in accord with her religious faith, insists on the provision of care because all life should be protected. A federal appeals court has ruled, by a 2-1 vote, that the hospital must treat the child for her apneic episodes, based on the Emergency Medical Treatment and Active Labor Act of 1986 (the "anti-dumping" act). The hospital currently is in the process of appealing the decision.

Although this scenario may be uncommon, it offers several points of discussion for the everyday practice of health care. For example, should patient or proxy autonomy carry equal weight when a treatment is being requested as opposed to being refused? What are the ethical obligations of physicians and hospitals to provide care they deem futile? Based on an "ethic of care," is the more caring approach to a case such as this to offer seemingly useless treatment to appease religious or other patient or proxy needs, especially when the treatment imposes no additional burdens on the patient? Finally, to what extent should the law influence and intervene in health care decision making?

Principles

Today the principle of autonomy significantly influences law and health care, perhaps inordinately. The principle rightly strives to protect a constitutive element of who we are as human beings—namely, our freedom and ability to choose. One interprets this autonomy in the context of a shared decision-making process that integrates patient values with medical expertise and knowledge that promotes the well-being of the patient. Certainly, when patients make informed and free decisions, based on their values and goals in life, to refuse certain treatments, such decisions are essentially sacrosanct even though the health care professional might not make the same choice. For instance, physicians honor an adult Jehovah's Witness patient's decision to forego a life-saving blood transfusion. We respect and accept the "negative" precept not to violate patient autonomy when refusal of treatment is involved. Does this negative right of refusal imply a positive right to demand and to be provided with any desired treatment? For the most part, requests for treatment are honored—though the obligation does not seem as binding as that of complying with a refusal of treatment, especially when the request violates principles of good medicine and the autonomy and values of the health care professional. Consequently, the health care professional's effort to respect patient autonomy does not always include the obligation to give the patient whatever treatment he or she desires. In some sense, this principle is self-evident in that a physician would not prescribe morphine for a simple headache because that was the patient's analgesic of choice or help kill a patient because of a request for euthanasia.

Discussion

In the case of Baby K, the refusal of doctors to acquiesce to the autonomous decision of the mother hinges on the assumption that the care being requested constitutes "futile" treatment. How is "futility" to be defined, and by whom? Baby K's mother may say that the respiratory treatments are not futile; they preserve the child's life: How can that be futile? Substituting terms such as nonbeneficial or ineffective for futile may help because they connote a notion of a lack of an ability to carry out human purposes. An effective or beneficial treatment must offer reasonable hope that the person can pursue goals or goods in life. In the case of Baby K— assuming the accuracy of the diagnosis and prognosis—her underlying anencephalic condition necessarily excludes that possibility. This linguistic alteration may not be foolproof, however, because some people would argue that treatments that preserve physiological life appear effective, especially if one's religious beliefs lead one to conclude that preservation of life is a worthwhile goal.

In commenting on the case, ethicist Robert Veatch cautioned physicians against making quality-of-life judgments and stressed that parents have equal expertise to make such decisions. Thus, the physicians should comply with the directives of Baby K's mother. Veatch correctly posits that in assessing the burdens of treatment, certain quality-of-life judgments are made wherein the physician has no particular expertise.

Does this case involve estimations of quality of life, or should we rightly speak of the estimation of quality of function? In determining the effectiveness of a treatment, a more objective medical standard prevails: quality of function. That is, in measuring effectiveness, one must assess if the treatment has the capacity to restore functional ability in the patient so that he or she can pursue cognitive/effective purposes. Physicians at times may lack the ability to make quality-of-life judgments that involve the patient's own values. They are eminently qualified, however, to make quality-of-function determinations. Although the number of cases in which the criteria for futility or ineffectiveness are satisfied may be limited, the case of Baby K is one of them.

In situations like the Baby K case, some people have recommended moving away from a principle-based method of ethical decision making wherein rules are applied dispassionately. Instead they offer an ethic of care. Such an ethic would speak of concern, compassion, and commitment. Rather than become embroiled in legal proceedings and discussions of quality of function, an ethic of care would gear itself toward supporting relationships—in case, that of mother and child. Futility would not be measured by the medical effect on the patient but by the effect on social relationships. Thus, even though the health care professional may believe the treatment to be inappropriate, an ethic of care might lead one to reason that there is no harm in continuing to treat, especially when religious beliefs are at stake. Is not discretion the better part of valor? Maximizing the patient's and surrogate's happiness takes precedence over that of the health care worker. One is called to do the "most caring" action.

An immediate weakness of such an approach is the issue of how we know what is the "most caring" thing to do. Certainly, everyone favors compassionate care in health care. We only discern what the caring thing to do is, however, by analyzing what it means to be a human being and developing principles and norms of conduct that are based on our basic needs. By ostensibly doing the caring thing in continuing to resuscitate the child, we may be creating more grief for the mother when the child eventually dies.

There are other significant harms associated with following a proxy's wishes to avoid confrontation. The danger exists that health care professionals will be transformed into technicians whose health care expertise would be reduced to minimal import in decision making, thereby distorting what it means to be a professional. In the case of Baby K, economic issues may also be involved. Even though the child has full insurance coverage, other policy holders will have to make up the difference eventually. Important as the financial issue is, it should not obscure the primary reason for removing or not offering treatment—namely, that the treatment is ineffective.

One of the most frustrating elements of the Baby K case is the court's involvement and its bizarre application of anti-dumping laws—which were never meant to apply to anencephalic children whose treatment is not warranted. Sadly, the erroneous assumption that underlies this court's decision is that medicine treats illnesses rather than persons affected by illness. It would have been easier to fathom the decision if the court had ordered the treatment to emphasize a nearly inviolable status of surrogate decision making. To further complicate matters, the law can be interpreted very idiosyncratically. In another state, a court might have adjudicated the case differently.

For better or for worse, legal interventions affect the treatment of patients. Sometimes the law legitimately protects and promotes the well-being of patients and health care workers. At other times (as in the case of Baby K), the law is a grossly inadequate means for resolving what are fundamentally ethical dilemmas. Unfortunately, court decisions, legislation, and the threat of criminal and civil suits can weaken the resolve of the most ethical health care professional.

What is a person to do? In very protracted cases, transferring the patient always remains a viable option. In the Baby K case, because of the emergency need for treatment and the reluctance of other facilities to take the child, such a transfer is contraindicated. Although an individual practitioner cannot be coerced into acting against his or her conscience by the law, until the case is appealed or the legislation amended, an institution as institution may have to capitulate. Even that action, however, may be a dangerous precedent to set when the law coerces an institution to do something morally repugnant. At what point would one draw the line?

Conclusion

The Baby K case has exasperated all parties concerned. Health care professionals may be tempted to compromise their beliefs and yield to inappropriate proxy demands. They may perceive this action as the "caring thing to do" and as a sound risk-management strategy, even though it would violate the standards of medical practice. That approach, however, subjects the field of health care to the whims of the law and relegates the health care worker to the status of technician rather than professional. To avoid that reality requires one to take a stand. Of course, such stands can be taken with pastoral sensitivity that try to enter into the pain and sorrow of the mother and try to ascertain why the mother refuses to let go. In cases such as this, the danger is that all parties may end up losing. The Baby K case indicates the extent to which unbridled autonomy, individualism, and the law have infiltrated the health care decision-making process. Is it time to take a stand, or is discretion still the better part of valor?

Part Four

Genetics

Chapter 39 _____

Cloning (Artificial Twinning): Have We Gone Too Far?

On October 26, 1993, the *New York Times* reported that Dr. Jerry Hall and colleagues at the George Washington University Medical Center had cloned human embryos. The subsequent firestorm of debate conjured up images of *Brave New World* and *Jurassic Park,* as well as the possibility of hundreds of Adolf Hitlers being created from residual hair from his head. The technology available today and well into the foreseeable future, however, would not allow for this type of cloning because human cells specialize very early in development. As some *Newsweek* pundits wrote: "A lock of Hitler's hair, even if scientists could extract its DNA, would only give rise to the world's most disgusting hairball."[1] Nevertheless, the artificial creation of twins by means of *in vitro* fertilization techniques in conjunction with cloning methods gives birth to numerous ethical questions.

The Techniques and Purposes of Cloning

The scientists performed their cloning experiments on embryos at various stages of development (up to the eight-cell stage). All of the embryos had genetic malformations because of penetration of the ovum by multiple sperm. Scientists treated these embryos with an enzyme to dissolve the protective shell (the zona pellucida) surrounding the embryonic cells. The identical cells were split apart chemically. The researchers then used sodium alginate to provide a new but artificial zona pellucida that allowed for the growth of the newly formed embryos. Some of the cloned embryos reached

145

the 32-cell stage of development before they were destroyed (scientists had no intention of implanting the defective embryos).

The main purpose of this type of research is to enhance the possibility that infertile couples will be able conceive via *in vitro* fertilization. Some infertile couples lack the ability to produce a large number of embryos for implantation. The success rate of implantation for each individual embryo is very low (the overall pregnancy rate is 5–15 percent). Therefore, by increasing the number of embryos implanted through cloning, scientists hope to increase the odds that infertile couples will bear children.

The cloning technology would have other applications. For example, scientists already have the ability to detect genetic defects in embryos at very early cellular development. However, techniques of analysis have an inherent risk of destroying the embryo. Cloning would provide an expendable embryo that could be analyzed and destroyed while its twin was safeguarded for implantation. Parents could also freeze cloned embryos and then choose to implant them later, after the first child has grown. This possibility leads to the theoretical but unlikely scenario that a woman could give birth to her own twin sister twenty-five years later. Parents could also preserve embryos for later implantation in case the first child dies or needs some type of transplant from an identical donor. This scenario may not be so far-fetched: Parents in California conceived a child solely for the purpose of providing bone marrow for their teenage daughter suffering from leukemia. In the currently unregulated field of reproductive technologies, one could envision a market for prospective parents who could choose embryos based on what the twin already looks like. Many years in the future, if genetic engineering becomes more refined, one could select for and produce multiple human beings with a particular trait.

Ethical Concerns

The technology of cloning and its application clearly raise many issues about human reproduction, individual identity, and the status of the embryo. Yet the discussion of such issues can be hindered because science and technology are considered distinct from ethics. Some people believe that science merely involves the pursuit of knowledge. This dissociation of the scientific researcher from ethics fails to recognize that because science affects human beings and their values, it must be an ethical endeavor—an endeavor that should not use scientific ends to justify the means, at the expense of human dignity. Hence, several worldwide ethical commissions from Germany, Australia, and Economic Summit countries have condemned any type of nontherapeutic research on embryos. Once more, we must examine critically science's impact on human life, especially that of embryos.

The most significant ethical issue surrounding cloning is the status of the embryo. In the United States, where scientists and the public cannot agree on the moral status and rights of the fetus, there certainly will be less respect for the rights of the embryo. As an indication of that likelihood, a popular magazine predicted that the new technique of blastomere analysis for genetic defects with subsequent discarding of defective embryos would avoid the moral dilemma of abortion and the destruction of human beings.

The underlying assumption present in that statement must be evaluated and challenged. Science has indicated that from the time of conception (when fusion of the maternal and paternal pro-nuclei is complete), the new life (as distinct from mother and father) self-directs its own development with some initial assistance of maternal cytoplasm. In interpreting these scientific facts, many people assert that the embryo represents more than a potential person but already a person with potential. Even in the absence of consensus about the interpretation of the scientific facts and the status of the embryo as a person, what does the deliberate destruction of "defective" embryos say to and for children who are born with diseases such as Tay-Sachs disease, Duchenne muscular dystrophy, or other birth anomalies? Thus, the protection of new life and the respect that should be accorded to all human beings seems to be lacking in the general discussion of cloning and many reproductive technologies.

Another fundamental issue attached to the technology of cloning is the conceptualization of our relationship with children. In contemporary society, the old maxim that children should be "seen and not heard" has yielded to a growing phenomenon of physical, sexual, and psychological abuse. In the United States, more than one-fifth of children live in poverty. Will cloning lead to further insensitivity toward children? Although one must be sensitive to infertile couples, reproductive technologies have suggested in many minds that parents have a right to children. In the process, children take on the status of objects to be possessed rather than subjects to be respected. Certainly, many infertile couples choose *in vitro* fertilization for loving and unselfish reasons. Yet embryos are discarded because of defects or, in some cases, simply because they are of the wrong sex. Cloning will probably only add to the affront to the dignity of children because couples may have even better means to genetically analyze their child before implantation. The embryos and children take on the semblance of products— or, as one Tennessee divorce case decided, quasi-property.

With this strong product metaphor, it is no wonder ethicists are concerned about the development of markets for embryos that would use them as means to an end. On a societal level, one must wonder whether cloning will provide a vehicle in the future for a negative eugenics movement. Although human beings as a whole believe they are beyond such behavior, xenophobia and ethnic cleansing in Europe should serve as a reminder that a certain unscrupulousness lurks in the depths of the human heart. Moreover, it raises the question about the long-range effect on the gene pool and the natural selection process if we select out for certain traits and make multiple copies of people with "desirable" traits.

Test-tube twinning may exacerbate existing problems associated with certain reproductive technologies. Besides the dilemmas associated with famous cases such as the Baby M surrogacy case, problems accrue on a daily basis as thousands of embryos today remain frozen in suspended animation, their fate undecided. Cloning will only add to those numbers. In an age of depersonalization of our sexual nature, cloning and asexual reproduction may contribute to the erosion of our sense of the gift of procreativity, our role as parents, the meaning of heritage, and our understanding of sexual intercourse and love. Finally, at a time when our country grapples with ways to provide basic health services to all, is cloning an appropriate and well founded line of investigation if millions of dollars will be devoted to helping only a relatively few individuals?

Conclusion

In the arena of science and technology, often one is either a technophile or technophobe. Neither position honestly and critically analyzes the advancement of science. To dismiss advances in genetics simply because they draw us closer to a brave new world denies our creative genius as human beings and our ability to improve our lifestyle. Likewise, to fail to assess the ethical nature and impact of science on humanity would deny the very nature of science itself, which necessarily affects the human community.

A critical assessment of cloning or artificial twinning reveals that it does not involve the exaggerated fears linked to best sellers such as *Jurassic Park*. Nevertheless, the cloning debate has yet to give proper weight to the status of the embryo. Although debate over the embryo will continue, the question we must ask is, Can we afford to be wrong when the life of an individual hangs in the balance? Moreover, the applications of cloning reflect an inadequate respect for the developing embryo and an unfortunate trend toward viewing the child as object and product rather than personal subject. Even the most innocuous use of cloning—to provide additional embryos to increase the chance of success of pregnancy—should cause us to reflect on the ethical acceptability of various reproductive technologies. As we enter this brave new world of science, society will need insightful women and men of great courage to act on behalf of the human community—especially the children.

Note

1. J. Adler, M. Hager, and K. Springen, "Clone Hype," *Newsweek,* November 18, 1993, 61.

Chapter 40

Genetic Testing: Ethics Issues

A wry friend claims that he likes to go to the meeting of the local genetics society because it makes him very optimistic about the state of his health. He states that when he went to the meeting ten years ago, he realized that his genetic makeup enabled him to avoid about five hundred diseases. Now, with new genetic information available, he maintains that his genetic makeup has enabled him to avoid 4,000 diseases—many of them fatal.

More and more information is available concerning our genetic make-up and the diseases that result from genetic malfunction. Much of this information is the result of the Human Genome Project. The Human Genome Project is also developing tools to identify the genes involved in these diseases. Molecular diagnosis has sparked a revolution in the diagnosis of genetic disorder. A molecular study can determine the presence or absence of gene mutation and thereby allow a diagnosis to be made well in advance of the appearance of clinical symptoms.

As a result of new genetic information, tests for genetic diseases are being developed—usually by for-profit pharmaceutical companies.

Presymptomatic testing clearly will be a significant factor in changing the emphasis in medical care. In the past, people sought the help of physicians after the onset of illness or disease. In the future, medical efforts will be directed toward preventive medicine—toward helping people avoid or mitigate the diseases for which they have a genetic predisposition. Not only will testing for diseases that may occur later change the practice of medicine; predictive pre-symptomatic testing is expected to become "a boom industry."[1]

Although presymptomatic testing is usually presented as just one more step in the battle against disease, several ethical issues arise from its use. A few of these ethical issues arising from genetic testing have been considered frequently. For example, it is well known that the release of genetic information can cause discrimination insofar as insurance and employment is concerned. This chapter presents some ethical questions about gene testing and genetic engineering that are considered less often.

Ethical Issues

When tests become available, we assume that the general public will be interested in utilizing them, depending upon the primary care physician to interpret them. This pattern certainly obtains with regard to tests recently developed to detect prostate cancer. Several facts make testing of the general public a questionable practice, however. First, there currently is no understanding of the false negatives and false positives that will occur.[2] Such errors are easier to avoid when testing is conducted in a meticulous research environment and restricted to people whose family history indicate that they are at risk. When testing moves beyond high-risk families, it becomes more complex. Even though a gene mutation often associated with cancer may be detected, insofar as the general public is concerned the mutation may not in fact be predictive for cancer. If a person belongs to a family with a history of early-onset cancer, a genetic mutation in itself is cause for concern. With regard to the general public, however, a mutation does not have the same import. To understand the meaning of a mutation in a member of the general public, "we need to develop functional assays in order to determine what a mutation means," says Rick Fiskel, a member of the team that pinpointed the genes that dispose for colon cancer.[3] We need much greater accuracy before gene testing for genetic disease will be a reliable proposition. Putting genetic tests on the market will certainly attract many people to utilize the tests who have little risk of cancer. Will this testing be beneficial, or will it merely increase questionable expenditures?

Another ethical issue concerns the need for counseling for those who seek genetic information. Counseling for people seeking genetic information is of two kinds: psychological counseling and genetic counseling. The need for psychological counseling arises when people wish to determine whether they are subject to fatal genetic disorders, such as Huntington's disease. Usually, people who request such testing have had relatives who have died from the disease. If the test is a true negative, the person will be relieved and the test may be considered "successful." If the test is a true positive, however, other issues are involved. The results of the test will not "save the person's life" because the mutative genes that give rise to the disease are already present. Will positive results be devastating for afflicted individuals? Good psychological counseling can help persons avoid severe depression. One long-term study of potential Huntington patients suggests the benefits of testing whether results are positive or negative, if accompanied by competent psychological testing.[4]

Genetic counseling is another question. Genetic counseling is essential to educate patients about genetics, about probabilities, about false negatives and false positives. At present, however, there are only about one thousand genetic counselors in the United States, most within university centers. The general population will seek help in interpreting genetic tests from their primary care physicians. "Most doctors have only the vaguest idea of the implication of genetic testing," says Bruce Ponder of Cambridge University, a member of the team that isolated the genes involved in breast cancer.[5] Is there hope that physicians will be able to achieve this knowledge? Although there are thorough courses in genetic theory in medical schools, little attention is given to the implication of genetic testing. Hence, sufficient opportunity for physicians to obtain this knowledge should be offered through continuing education programs to enable physicians to address the ethical issues that might result from inaccurate counseling.

The question that has puzzled me for some time is whether genetic mutations are really errors in the long run. Given the knowledge that we are all mortal beings and that we share in a common genetic inheritance, are we really making progress for society as a whole if we eliminate the effects of individual genetic mutations? Jared Diamond raised this point a few years ago when he discussed the tendency of Ashkenazic Jews to develop Tay-Sachs disease as a result of a genetic disposition to accumulate fats.[6] Diamond suggests that many common diseases may persist because they bring blessings as well as curses. If a person inherits two copies of a faulty gene, the person may die or be seriously impaired as a result. However, if a person inherits only one gene—that is, if he or she is a carrier of the genetic disease but not a victim of it—the one defective gene may protect the person against other diseases. Diamond notes that persons who are carriers of the Tay-Sachs gene seem to be protected from tuberculosis, even though they have lived at times and places when tuberculosis was common. Whatever the value of the foregoing consideration, our genetic inheritance clearly has a social dimension as well as a personal effect. Will the gene pool for future generations be affected by efforts to eliminate genes that are harmful for individuals?

Moreover, who will benefit from genetic testing? Will it be confined to those who have health care coverage? Will genetic testing and the ability to combat some future genetic anomaly be available to uninsured persons? Underlying every advance in health care technology should be the realization that more than forty million people in the United States have limited access to health care. This statistic is the basis for a petition signed by several religious leaders to prohibit the current practice of allowing commercial corporations to patent human genes and genetically engineer animals, thus putting these valuable sources of health and well-being beyond the reach of many people.

Finally, in the future, how will we look upon those who have genetic defects? At present, we tend to sympathize with people who have genetic defects and offer compassionate care. We subsidize the care of genetically debilitated persons through home health care or institutional care. In the future, however, will we be as concerned about people with disabilities if we think their disabilities could have been avoided? The information resulting from genetic studies may enable researchers to develop cures for some fatal diseases. Yet the increase in genetic information and genetic therapy will change the way we relate to one another. Our attitudes toward life, death, disability, and suffering will change. Do we have the wisdom to use our newfound knowledge and technology to improve the well-being of all?

Conclusion

An old Irish proverb states, "If you want to see God smile, tell him your plans." In other words, our new genetic knowledge and technology should be developed and applied carefully.

Notes

1. R. Nowak, "Genetic Testing Set to Take Off," *Science*, July 22, 1994, 464.

2. National Center for Genome Research, "Human Genome Project: From Maps to Medicine" (Washington, D.C.: National Institutes of Health, 1995).
3. Nowak, "Genetic Testing Set to Take Off," 465.
4. Law Reform Commission, "Canadian Collaborative Study of Predictive Testing," 1992.
5. Nowak, "Genetic Testing Set to Take Off," 465.
6. J. Diamond, "Curse and Blessing of the Ghetto," *Discover,* March 1991, 60–66.

Chapter 41 _____

Concerns about Genetic Testing: Is a Little Knowledge Dangerous?

In a *Time* magazine poll, only 50 percent of people responded affirmatively to the following question: "If it were possible, would you want to take a genetic test telling you which diseases you are likely to suffer from later in life?"[1] The expansion of genetic knowledge and the development of predictive genetic tests creates a set of dilemmas for patients wherein two traditional maxims sum up many people's viewpoint: "Ignorance is bliss," and "A little knowledge is dangerous." Would we prefer to be blissfully ignorant and not know that a time-bomb lurks in the recesses of our genetic make-up—ready to explode in a year, five years, ten years, or perhaps forty years? If individuals were to have access to this genetic knowledge, could decisions surrounding treatment, lifestyle changes, and social policy threaten their well-being?

A Framework of Analysis

As with any technology, an ethical analysis of our ability to predict disease based on a genetic profile begins and ends with the question, How does the technology and its use promote the well-being of persons and society as a whole? In addition, we must ask, What presumptions about the nature of disease and human anthropology do we make? What respective roles do genetics and the environment play in our health status? The "nature versus nurture" debate takes on even greater importance when we delve into the genetics of behavior and intelligence—for example, the alleged connection between genetics and criminal behavior.

Raising the Issues

Beyond those critical contextual questions lie more practical concerns with regard to genetic testing of patients. How accurate are the tests—that is, what are the percentages of false negatives and positives? What meaning do the predictive tests have? For example, the person who tests positive for the Huntington's disease gene will eventually manifest the disease because of the autosomal dominant nature of the condition. The test will not necessarily predict, however, when the disease will strike. An even more complicated situation emerges when genetic analysis indicates only a predisposition toward a particular condition such as heart disease or colon or breast cancer. How does one interpret such probabilities? An affected person may have a relative risk that is several times greater than that of the general population, but what does that fact mean if the risk for the general population is very low to begin with? Even lifetime cumulative risks (e.g., a 50 percent chance of developing a disease) do not always specify when the disease will be manifested. Nor can one always predict to what extent the genes will be expressed symptomatically (a concept known as incomplete penetrance).

Another set of questions focuses on the benefits and burdens of genetic knowledge. Unfortunately, a concomitant burden often is attached to each of the benefits. As an illustration of this fact, consider three issues. First, identification of conditions such as familial hypercholesterolemia or adenomatous polyposis (which predisposes one toward colon cancer) may allow for lifestyle alterations and/or more aggressive monitoring of the patient to prevent symptomatic manifestation of the disease or to treat it in its earliest stages. In cases in which one only has a predisposition toward a disease, however, one may be accepting the risks associated with treatments for a disease that one may never develop. Whereas minor interventions (e.g., dietary alterations) might be instituted for a person with a fairly low predisposition toward heart disease or diabetes, one would require a higher probability of developing a disease to justify a prophylactic mastectomy or oophorectomy. How can we determine when a statistical probability warrants intervention?

Second, based on family histories, at-risk individuals may desire to know their status for the sake of peace of mind. On the downside, in situations for which no current treatment exists, individuals receiving positive results must live with the psychologically stressful knowledge of the impending manifestation of the disease. Even individuals who receive negative results often experience survivor's guilt. Moreover, a negative result could lull individuals into a false sense of security. For instance, more than 90 percent of women who develop breast cancer do not test positive for the breast cancer gene (BRCA1). Third, knowledge of one's carrier status for particular genetic diseases may assist couples in making decisions about conceiving children. Many genetic diseases exhibit a later onset, however. Should one choose not to conceive because the person will develop Huntington's at the age of 40 or 50? How does our current expectation of life-span prejudice our answer to the question? Moreover, what statistical probability of passing on a severely deleterious trait should warrant the avoidance of conception (1/2, 1/4, 1/10)? To what extent should society be involved in that decision, if at all?

As with many bioethical decisions involving burden and benefit, one must qualitatively assess seemingly incommensurate goods. Colloquially, one must compare apples and oranges. Consider the 36-year-old woman with a significant family history of breast cancer who possesses the BRCA1 gene. More frequent mammograms and breast exams may help to detect the cancer earlier; reliable data about the efficacy of such monitoring, however, is not yet available given the recent discovery of the gene. Yet the woman also lives daily with the knowledge that she has a 20 percent chance to develop cancer by age 40, a 50 percent risk to develop cancer by the age of 50, and an 85 percent lifetime risk, whereas women in general have an 11 percent lifetime risk of breast cancer. Consequently, some women opt for a more definitive cure through prophylactic radical bilateral mastectomy. Yet this choice has implications for the woman's self-identity, in addition to the risks associated with surgery. Moreover, for a small percentage of women, prophylactic surgery does not absolutely guarantee eradication of the possibility of cancer because it can develop in the chest wall. Finally, there is a cost factor. Currently, insurers are reluctant to pay for prophylactic surgeries and breast reconstruction. No wonder Lisa Parker summarizes the conflicting feelings and ambivalence of women who see their breasts "as time bombs that they desperately want to diffuse, but do not want to be rid of."[2] Given the patient-specific effects of the decision, physicians generally should trust the subjective decisions of women in these cases. Yet at what point does the risk not justify a preventive mastectomy?

Confidentiality and Social Concerns

The use of genetic testing gives rise to confidentiality concerns. Should an individual's genetic conditions be shared with a fiancee, spouse, children, employers, insurance companies, or the government? Although individuals may have a moral duty to share some genetic information with their family, the physician would not have an ethical obligation to divulge information about patients unless the condition created a serious and imminent physical danger to a third party. Unlike traditionally reportable information about child abuse, sexually transmitted diseases, and gunshot wounds, failure to disclose genetic information usually poses no direct threat of physical harm to a third party.

Greater confidentiality concerns arise when employers and insurers have access to such information. The Americans with Disabilities Act restricts employment discrimination on the basis of genetic makeup unless it directly applies to job performance. We should not be so naive, however, as to presume that knowledge of a costly genetic condition or carrier status will not lead to more covert forms of discrimination, particularly in terms of insurance (especially for self-insured employers). Under certain circumstances, insurers might try to deny coverage, raise rates to exorbitant levels, or deny payment for treatment of symptoms because they involved pre-existent genetic conditions. Recognition of the right to health care and the provision of basic access would ameliorate many of these concerns. For now, however, government regulations will have to continue to close some of the loopholes on such discrimination.

Widespread development and dissemination of genetic testing will generate resource allocation questions. Based on cost effectiveness, should widespread screening be employed (e.g., as is currently done with PKU), or should testing be done on a restricted population of high-risk individuals? Should people who are not high risk have access to testing? Moreover, who or what is driving the movement toward increased testing: Is it legitimate patient need or biotech companies that stand to make large profits—or both? Who will monitor quality control? As demand for testing grows, there may not be a sufficient number of highly trained genetic counselors to advise patients. Will general practitioners be able to discuss the complexities of genetics and genetic therapy when it becomes more commonplace?

Conclusion

The uses for and utilization of genetic testing will continue to expand. Given the complexity of the science of genetics and the prevalence of misunderstanding by the lay public, physicians must be scrupulous about obtaining true informed consent when they perform genetic tests. Patients must understand the pros and cons of testing. They must be able to assimilate the nature of genetic disease. They must understand the reliability of the information and be able to put the probabilities associated with the diseases into the context of their lives. They must be aware of options other than testing, as well as options once testing is done. Finally, physicians must verify that individuals are not unduly coerced into poor treatment decisions by irrational fears of genetic disease. Genetic testing holds much promise for the health status of individuals and society. Until many of the foregoing questions are answered, however, genetic testing may involve significant peril.

Notes

1. P. Elmer-Dewitt, "The Genetic Revolution," *Time* (January 17, 1994), 50. The affirmative percentage increases substantially if there is a familial history of disease.
2. L. Parker, "Breast Cancer Genetic Screening and Critical Bioethics' Gaze," *Journal of Medicine and Philosophy* 20 (June 1995), 329.

Chapter 42 _____

Cloning Human Beings

On July 5, 1996, animal researchers at Edinburgh's Roslin Institute disclosed that they had successfully transferred genetic material from the cell of an adult sheep into another sheep's egg (with its genetic material removed), implanting the resulting embryo in a third sheep that gave birth to a lamb named Dolly. Prior to the birth of Dolly, scientists had believed that once adult cells differentiated—to become skin cells or eye cells, for example—their DNA would no longer be usable to form a mammal. Dolly, however, is the "delayed" genetic twin of a single adult mammal. Chicago physicist Richard Seed has proposed to use the same cloning technique, called somatic cell nuclear transfer (SCNT), to create a child. On January 6, 1998, Seed announced that he plans to offer the option of cloning to infertile couples who wish to have a child. At this time it is not clear whether the FDA will assume jurisdiction over Seed's research. If so, he will likely set up his private, for-profit "Human Clone Clinic" outside the United States.

Much of the initial reaction to Seed's announcement has been negative, although often without clear articulation about exactly what makes us uncomfortable. People express fears about the potential harms to children who may be created by cloning—particularly psychological harms associated with a diminished sense of individuality and uniqueness. Others worry about the effect on parenting and family relationships. Immediately after the report of the cloning of Dolly, President Clinton barred federal funding related to attempts to clone human beings (with allowance for some research to clone embryos that would not be implanted) and requested voluntary compliance from researchers in the private and nonfederally funded sectors. Seed claims that he is not bound by these prohibitions because he is a private researcher who happens to disagree with the president's stance on cloning. Being clear about human cloning is the first step in understanding why it matters morally and whether it differs from other assisted reproductive technologies, such as *in vitro* fertilization (IVF).

Human Cloning Technology

There are two distinct ways in which SCNT from an adult differs from other assisted-reproduction technologies. First, SCNT goes beyond current forms of artificial reproduction, which have been performed using both egg and sperm. It replaces sexual procreation with asexual replication of an existing set of genes from a single adult. Cloning removes insemination and fertilization from the marriage relationship, and it can completely eliminate one of the partners from the reproductive process. Second, SCNT makes it possible to predetermine the genes of a child. The prospective parent(s) would know in advance a great deal about their child's genetic characteristics. This tremendously increased power to control the genetic makeup of our children raises moral concerns about individuality and human dignity. Psychologist Sidney Callahan argues that the random fusion of a couple's genetic heritage allows the child to be seen as a separate other; even identical twins have different genetic blueprints than their parents.

Consider the following scenarios—one related to human cloning and the other to IVF. In the first scenario, an infertile married couple decides that

SCNT is the best technology to create the child they desire. The mother's egg and the genetic material from one of her cells are used to create an embryo (outside the womb), which is implanted in the mother. She gives birth to a child who has her genetic make-up only. In the second scenario, the same couple elects to pursue IVF. The mother's egg and father's sperm is fertilized by the (outside the womb), and the resulting embryo is implanted in the mother. She gives birth to a child who has the genetic make-up of both parents. In both situations, "extra" embryos may be destroyed or frozen for later use. Dolly was cloned after 276 unsuccessful attempts; some developing embryos had to be eliminated because of genetic abnormalities and other DNA problems that made them unsuitable for implantation.

The widespread use of IVF indicates that it is socially, although not necessarily ethically, acceptable in our society. Our acceptance of most assisted reproductive technologies may mean that we have effectively dismissed the moral arguments that would also apply to cloning persons. Perhaps safety and efficacy are the only moral issues left to us. The profound issues raised by the potential for human cloning—perhaps the most extreme reproductive technology—prompt an evaluation of the following issues: (1) a ban on human cloning with the intent to create a child; (2) our ethical obligations to children; (3) the harmony between the demands of scientific inquiry and indispensable human values.

Discussion

First, we must determine why we would ban human cloning if we do not prohibit other reproductive technologies, such as IVF. Our visceral discomfort with human cloning, our concerns about dignity and using children as objects, and our unresolved questions about safety and efficacy may be sufficient reasons to call a moratorium. To be effective, however, a ban should include all cloning technologies with the intent of creating a child, as well as cloning research that would destroy human embryos. Some researchers want to perfect the cloning technique by creating embryos that would be discarded if they were unsuitable. The duration of a ban must also be considered. People who believe that human cloning is unacceptable in any circumstances will argue for a permanent ban. Those who believe that cloning might be acceptable in some circumstances (to provide a compatible source for bone marrow; to overcome infertility; to prevent genetic diseases) tend to favor a temporary ban or stricter regulation. In our pluralistic society, it may be possible to attain consensus only on a temporary ban at this time.

Second, we have an ethical obligation not to harm or impose serious risks on the children who would be created. Even if one believes that human cloning is morally licit in exceptional circumstances, the use of SCNT and other cloning techniques to create a child is premature and would expose the child to unknown, unacceptable risks. We do not have adequate data from research studies regarding the prospective safety and efficacy of cloning techniques in animals, much less in human beings. Even if we were to resolve the safety issues, however, there are other fundamental ethical concerns at stake. For example, although there are many warnings about the potential hazards to individual children, there are few reflections on how cloning might respond to the needs of future generations. No one yet has suggested that cloning would contribute to the flourishing of children or to the good of the adult whose genetic material is cloned.

Third, although we do not want to chill research that may produce future benefits, there are appropriate limits on scientific inquiry. In the face of a stunning scientific feat—such as cloning the first mammal—there is strong pressure to race forward with research. Scientists tell us that continued research using SCNT may result in skin issue for burn victims and organs for transplants. One of the primary goals of animal cloning is to make precise genetic changes in cells so animals could produce medicinal substances. Yet we do not have to accept uncritically the claim that cloning is a morally good way to reproduce or improve human beings. Since 1983, the European parliament and all the laws passed in Europe to legalize forms of artificial reproduction have forbidden human cloning. We can promote research that protects animals and plants and respects the biodiversity of species while prohibiting research on cloning with the intent of creating a child.

Conclusion

Albert Einstein observed that perfection of means and confusion of ends seem to characterize our age. The availability of cloning technology does not mean that the application to human beings is morally acceptable. A human being is not so much a genotype as a life journey; technology should be at the service of that human journey. Given the need for continued public discourse about the implications of human cloning, a ban on human cloning seems appropriate. Cloning of human persons should be banned not just because it is currently unsafe or because it is an extreme form of artificial reproduction, however, but because it denies the dignity of the human person as well as the dignity of human procreation.

Part Five

Organ Donation

Chapter 43

Organ Donation: Priceless Gift or Market Commodity?

More than 2,000 people die in the United States annually awaiting a suitable organ for transplantation. Moreover, every 20 minutes a new name is added to the list of people waiting for a kidney transplant. As the success of organ transplantation has increased, so has the demand for organs. Yet the supply of donors has remained relatively constant over the past five years. Although estimates vary, only about 20 percent of potential cadaver donors actually end up being donors.[1]

Recent efforts to maximize the retrieval of cadaveric organs have not succeeded. Required request laws that mandate that families of all potential donors be notified of the option to donate have been ineffective. Presumed consent—wherein it is presumed the person would want to donate one's organs unless specified otherwise—has been rejected as a viable alternative in the United States and has met with only limited success in Europe. In the United States, one untried solution to increase the supply of available organs is to create a market that provides incentives for donation. The buying and selling of organs initially strikes us as reprehensible and ghoulish on an emotional level. The National Organ Transplant Act of 1984 prohibits the acquisition, reception, and transfer of human organs for valuable consideration or payment as it affects interstate commerce laws. Several states have enacted similar legislation. Is there a concomitant ethical basis for proscribing the element of financial compensation in the field of organ procurement?

Living Donors

To facilitate the ethical analysis, one should divide the potential market into two types: a market for organs from living donors and one for organs from cadavers (the purchase of fetal tissue and organs from induced abortion are not considered here because of the intrinsic conflict of interest between the mother and the fetus). Recent stories from Latin America and India, where poor people sell kidneys to rich transplant recipients, have aroused moral outrage and condemnations of exploitation. Yet justifications for such behavior are frequently offered. First, supply is increased. Second, the donors receive compensation for their organs—which can sometimes be an economic lifesaver. Third, autonomy is enhanced as individuals exercise their liberty to use and dispose of their bodies as they see fit. Finally, people sell blood and other bodily products, so why not organs?

The first two arguments are strictly consequentialist. The merits of such arguments are debated on an empirical basis. The commercialization of organ procurement might result in a net decrease of available organs because it might increase suspicion of the transplant field. Furthermore, persons who would give altruistically might be offended by the commercialization of the "gift of life." Even if supply were to increase, however, would such good ends justify the means to them? Is there something inherently problematic with this practice? The sale of organs appears to be an act of financial desperation by poor people. The money offered as an enticement to donate is so coercive that it influences the individual unduly. This situation precludes the possibility of obtaining informed consent. Freedom is so compromised in such a case that true consent is not possible.

One might argue that we do not prevent poor from accepting more hazardous jobs, so why should we prohibit the removal of kidneys if it does not pose too great a risk? Two distinctions might be helpful. First, people have the freedom to leave a job at any time, whereas the removal of a kidney is a permanent procedure. Second, although work cannot be reduced to a transaction because it also pertains to an essential aspect of fulfillment for the human person, there is an inherently appropriate connection between work and just compensation for services rendered. To apply such an analogy to organ donation reduces the person to a commodity, a property composed of various body parts. Courtney Campbell comments that reducing ourselves to this status "expresses estrangement from our embodied experience."[2] We not only have stewardship over our bodies, we also "are our bodies."

This analysis explains why the selling of blood products does not repulse us, whereas the selling of organs does. Traditionally, people have argued that one can sell blood products because the sale presents no risks and the blood is a renewable source—whereas organs are not. The issue goes much deeper, however. When we sell the pint of blood, we do not perceive the body as being affected. When an organ is removed, however, one knows that one's body is being affected.

Thus, the only acceptable motivation for live donation has been charity. Whereas the selling of body parts for money alienates us from ourselves, altruistic donation reaches deeply into the meaning of personhood. As creatures directed to share our love, we fulfill that desire to be charitable through organ donation. Therefore, we perceive the selling of organs as reprehensible, whereas we regard charitable donation as courageous and magnanimous.

Cadaver Sources of Organs

Can the same reasoning be applied to the case of cadaveric sources of organs? In the case of cadaver donation, the problems of risk, coercion, and lack of consent are conspicuously absent. As a result, a more concerted effort to introduce financial inducements has been adopted. Could a market mechanism be established that is neither offensive nor easily abused? Most people would agree that it seems callous, offensive, and grossly utilitarian to approach grieving survivors and offer direct payment for their loved one's organs. The body is not distinct from the person; treating the body so blatantly as a commodity, as a collection of parts, offends the memory of the person.

Could more subtle and indirect forms of remuneration be more acceptable and less offensive? Indirect market methods of compensation might include paying the funeral costs for the family; offering a type of life insurance program in which beneficiaries would be reimbursed after donation; reducing health insurance premiums; waiving driver's license fees in exchange for signing the donor card; and even creating a futures market. Proponents argue that creating such incentives to promote donation benefits all. The corpse would not be harmed. Needy individuals will receive organs. People will receive compensation. In fact, not to do this would seem unethical because many people are condemned to death because of the lack of organs. Naturally, it would be better for people to give out of pure altruism. If such is not the case, however, why not provide an incentive?

Various arguments are offered in response to such reasoning. From a practical standpoint, such an approach again might be counterproductive because it might decrease altruistic donation. Additionally, payment for organs would increase the cost of an already expensive technology, especially if an open market were to develop. Finally, minorities and the poor might be further alienated from the system because they might feel they were being paid to provide organs for the rich.

On a more symbolic level, even after death a transcendent relationship remains between the person and the body. The corpse is not just decaying matter or property. Although our language sometimes refers to the body as property, especially in law, one should not assume that a similar terminology is philosophically appropriate. Relatives do not own the body of the deceased as if it were property or even quasi-property. Instead, they exercise respectful and dignified stewardship over the body because of their intrinsic link to the person and the obligations due that person as a member of the human community.

Admittedly, the buying of cadaver organs does not harm the deceased per se. Yet there may be considerable potential for harm to the human community from the undermining of our sense of altruism and compassion. By moving away from the concept of organ donation as gift, one transforms the body and ultimately the person into commodity and property. The more market-oriented the inducement strategy, the greater the assault to the dignity of the person. The general public's apprehension of the commercialization of organ donation should not be ignored. Although this intuitional moral sense that operates in the realm of symbol sometimes is dismissed as inexact and nebulous, it can arouse the conscience and direct us to the moral good.

Conclusion

The buying and selling of organs from living donors seems inappropriate. Although providing subtle financial inducements such as helping to pay funeral expenses in exchange for cadaveric organs is not clearly intrinsically wrong, the consequences of such an approach may not have the desired effects and may distort our vision of the human person. Given the gravity of the issue and the lives at stake, further discussion is needed in the area of cadaveric donation to clarify our understandings of life and death, body and property. Is "gift" the only paradigm in which to understand organ donation? Can one conceptually juxtapose self-centered and altruistic motivations in the same action? If more than 70 percent of U.S. citizens believe in donation, we should exhaust other alternatives before giving further consideration to the sale of cadaver organs. For example, reexamining the concept of presumed consent and encouraging compliance with required request laws by means of additional education and training may help.

Unfortunately, the numbers indicate that supply may never meet demand. Therefore, we may need to deal with the harder issue of reducing demand rather than increasing supply. Ultimately, will we have to reassess the technology in light of all of the other important goods of health care that remain unfulfilled today?

Notes

1. There are about 4,500 actual organ donors from 20,000–25,000 deaths from which organs could be procured. R. W. Evans et al. suggest that the number of potential donors may be at most 11,000. See "The Potential Supply of Organ Donors: An Assessment of the Efficacy of Organ Procurement Efforts in the United States." *JAMA* 267 (1992): 239–46.
2. C. Campbell, "Body, Self, and the Paradigm of Property," *Hastings Center Report* 22 (September–October, 1992), 42.

Chapter 44

Baby Theresa: "The Good That Could Be Done"

While Laura Campo and Justin Pearson awaited the birth of their baby, prenatal tests determined early in the pregnancy that the developing fetus suffered from anencephaly—a condition in which the higher centers of the brain fail to develop. Laura and Justin were aware that their baby, when born, would not survive because of this condition. They decided, however, to allow the pregnancy to go to term in hopes of donating their baby's organs to other newborns in need of them. When their baby Theresa was born, a dispute arose with regard to harvesting her organs.

When an anencephalic infant dies, the cause of death can range from hypoventilation and blood pressure instabilities to endocrine abnormalities and infection.[1] Depending on the manner in which death occurs, the infant's organs may not be suitable for transplantation. Fearing that their baby's organs would be rendered useless if she were allowed to die of natural causes, Theresa's parents sought to have her "declared" dead. Their request was prompted by physicians and others who argued that adhering to the current criteria for determining death causes precious organs to be wasted. Baby Theresa, however, was a living human being because she had a functioning brain stem that maintained integrated human function (albeit at a low level). Therefore, the proposal to declare her dead before her brain stem stopped functioning was a proposal to kill her.

It was obvious from media reports that Theresa's parents were caring persons who neither desired nor intended to harm their child. What, then, prompted such a request? Theresa's parents, like the parents of other anencephalic infants, suffered a great personal tragedy in bearing a child that is "born dying." The desire to find some meaning in the midst of such suffering can lead parents to accept as appropriate the proposal to change the criteria for defining when death has occurred.

Proposals to change current brain death criteria often reflect one or more of the following assumptions: (1) Because the anencephalic infant lacks the capacity for neocortical function, the anencephalic infant is not a person; (2) only persons should be considered to be alive, and current brain death criteria should be revised to reflect this; (3) using the anencephalic infant's organs for transplantation can "make sense" of a senseless situation; and (4) changing the criteria for determining death would avert the waste of valuable resources that could be used to save the lives of many other infants. This chapter explores these assumptions in order to support the conclusions that (a) the anencephalic infant is a living human being and should not be killed; (b) changing the present criteria for brain death would do nothing to alter the reality of when human death occurs and would serve only to sanction the killing of the infant in order to harvest organs; and (c) the desire to temper present suffering should not overcome the ability to make reasoned, ethical decisions about the appropriate care of an anencephalic infant.

Assessing the Assumptions

In a utilitarian attempt to maximize the greater good by making more organs available for transplantation, some people have argued that an anencephalic infant does not meet the criteria for human personhood. They maintain that because the cerebral cortex is absent and the infant lacks the capacity for personal activity, the infant should be "declared" dead and the organs harvested. The lack of present or future capacity for personal activity, however, does not change the fact that the infant is a living human being. The brain stem continues to regulate respiratory and cardiac function. Moreover, "because the neural structures that mediate typical newborn behaviors are located mainly in the brainstem, those anencephalic infants with relatively intact brainstems exhibit many such behaviors."[2]

In addition, attempts to determine a marker event or process (e.g., development of the cerebral cortex) delineating a difference between the human person and the human being consistently have failed.[3] Continued attempts to make such a distinction suggest that for some persons, basic human rights such as the right to life are not inherent and inalienable but conferred or earned once certain conditions have been met. One troubling conclusion from this kind of analysis is that the inability to meet the qualifying criteria render our responsibilities to the still-living human being null and void. Yet reason, supported by medical data, demands that the requirement that death be declared only when the whole brain—that is the cerebral cortex *and* the brain stem—ceases to function should be maintained. Moreover, our regard for the still-living, though debilitated, infant requires that we refrain from killing regardless of the motivation. On the other hand, because of the lack of potential for development of higher-level functions, we should not seek to prolong the anencephalic infant's life by the inappropriate use of life-sustaining interventions.

Although this analysis supports the appropriateness of maintaining current brain death criteria, it does nothing to mitigate the suffering experienced by the parents of the anencephalic infant. Nor does it address the appropriateness of trying to "make sense of the tragedy" by changing the rules to allow for killing to make the infant's organs available for transplantation. Here, two further considerations are important.

First, the desire to overcome the sense of helplessness and hopelessness that accompany the diagnosis and subsequent birth of an anencephalic infant is quite understandable. "These parents want something good to come from their tragedy; they want their child's life to have 'meaning' and the normal and healthy organs of their child to live on."[4] Yet the meaning or value of human life does not depend on functional or productive potential. The good of the human and its meaning are inherent in the human *as* human. This conviction is certainly contrary to the broader societal tendency to assign personal and social worth commensurate with the ability to produce or contribute to others and/or to society.

Second, the proposal to use the infant's organs to help the parents find some measure of solace in their grief shifts the focus of attention from the needs of the dying infant to the needs of the parents. Although parental needs are important, the infant is and must remain the primary patient. Appropriate care for the anencephalic infant entails providing things necessary for comfort and allowing death to come. If, after the infant's death, the organs are adequate for transplantation, they may be used. In addition, the reality of the parents' suffering demands not that the infant be "used" in attempts to "make sense" of their experience. Instead, the parents should be helped to appreciate the inherent good of life, to accept their loss and prepare for the approaching death of their child.

Some people would argue that such an approach is passive and too readily gives in to the inevitability of death. To the contrary, such an approach recognizes that human death is a natural part of life and that not every means to overcome the limits associated with human life is consistent with human good or well-being.

Finally, the enthusiasm of people who favor use of the anencephalic infant's organs for transplantation as a means of saving the lives of other infants must be tempered by reality. Medical data indicate that very few of the anencephalic infants born each year are acceptable as organ donors. Media coverage of cases like baby Theresa's, however, raise false hopes by noting that "about 5,000 children need pediatric organ transplants every year." Such statements are followed by the claim that "anencephalic babies are perfect donors."[5] Nowhere, however, is mention made of the fact that among the estimated 1,200 anencephalic infants born each year the usable kidneys, hearts and livers number 0, 69, and 61, respectively.[6]

Conclusion

The case of baby Theresa raises issues associated with human suffering, limitation, and death. As we continue to formulate individual and societal responses to these issues, we must keep in mind that expediency should not be allowed to overcome our willingness and ability to make sound ethical and medical judgments. The needs of the dying infant and the grieving parents require careful and compassionate consideration that aims to promote the good of both.

Notes

1. D. Alan Shewmon, "Anencephaly: Selected Medical Aspects," *Hastings Center Report* 18 (October/November 1988), 13.
2. Ibid.
3. President's Commission for the Study of Ethical Problems in Medicine and Research, *Defining Death* (Washington, D.C.: U.S. Government Printing Office, 1981), 39–40.
4. S. Ashwal et al., "Considerations of Anencephalic Infants as Organ Donor," *Biolaw* 2 (January 1992): 763–69.
5. "Baby Born without Brain Dies, But Legal Struggle Will Continue," *New York Times*, March 31, 1992.
6. D. Alan Shewmon et al., "The Use of Anencephalic Infants as Organ Sources," *JAMA* 261 (12): 1774.

Chapter 45 _____

The Baby Fae Legacy

Baby Fae was the first infant to receive a transplant of a baboon heart. Although she lived just short of three weeks with the transplant, the medical treatment she received spawned a host of ethical questions that live after her. This chapter considers some of these questions.

Principles

Most physicians and scientists in the United States doing research involving human subjects follow regulations for ethical research published by agencies of the federal government. Indeed, if the research in question is funded by the federal government, following the federal regulations is mandatory. Evaluation of human research protocols to ensure conformity with federal regulations is the responsibility of an institutional review board (IRB). An IRB, which is required at every research institution, is mainly concerned with protecting the human subjects involved in research projects; it also has some concern with the scientific validity of the project. At some schools—Saint Louis University, for example—all research projects involving human subjects must be approved by the IRB, not only those funded by the federal government.

The federal regulations for research involving children envision two types of research: research that "holds out prospects of direct benefit for the individual subject" and research that "does not hold out the prospect of direct benefit for the individual subject."[1] In the latter type of research, there may be a benefit resulting from the study—such as new scientific knowledge—that would benefit other children, but there is no direct benefit for the child or children involved in the research project. Concerning the first type of research, which involves therapeutic treatment for the child or children in question, the regulations for ethical research are similar to those regulating research on adult human subjects. Hence, consent must be received (in this case proxy consent because the child cannot give informed consent), and the risk of harm envisioned must be justified by the anticipated benefit.

With regard to research on children who do not benefit directly, however, the regulations are more involved. First, a distinction is made between "minimal risk of harm" to the subject and "more than minimal risk of harm." *Minimal risk* is equivalent to "physical and psychological harm that is normally encountered in the daily lives or in the routine medical or psychological examination of healthy children." Research that involves *more than* minimal risk may be approved by the IRB if there is "only a *minor increase* over minimal risk" and other requirements are met. If the IRB finds that the research involves a *major increase* over minimal risk, "the IRB can refer the project to the Department of Health and Human Services for study by a panel of experts," provided the IRB also "finds that the research presents a reasonable opportunity to further the understanding, prevention or alleviation of a serious problem affecting the health and welfare of children."

Some ethicists believe that the federal regulations for research involving children are too lenient insofar as nonbeneficial research is concerned. The main reason for this disagreement lies in the nature of proxy consent. A parent or guardian has the right of proxy consent only to benefit his or her child or ward. Although an adult may freely subject himself or herself to risk research in which there is no personal benefit, a parent or guardian does not have the same right over a child. Whatever the value of this opinion, the treatment given Baby Fae was unethical even in light of the more liberal ethical norms contained in the federal regulations.

Discussion

To offer an ethical evaluation, we pose the following questions:

- Should the physicians who performed the transplant on Baby Fae have followed the federal guidelines for research on children? Legally speaking, they did not have to follow these guidelines because the research was funded by withholding a portion of the fees collected from private patients. (This method of funding research is an ethical issue in itself because cost shifting is involved.) Morally speaking, though, the researchers at Loma Linda University do appear to have an obligation to follow the federal regulations because they offer minimal ethical standards for our pluralistic society. In other words, if researchers do not follow the federal norms, which ethical norms will they follow?

- Did this research benefit Baby Fae directly, or did it offer the kind of knowledge that would benefit other children? Despite some early enthusiastic statements from some of the physicians doing the transplant, there seems to be no doubt that the transplant was not of direct benefit to Baby Fae. Some people might say, "Baby Fae benefited because she would have died anyway, and the transplant prolonged her life." Research may never be justified, however, simply because the subject "will die anyway." Moreover, what benefit is it to prolong the life of an infant for three weeks and treat the infant as a thing rather than a person during that time? Others might say, "Maybe by some miracle she could have lived." Scientific research on human beings is not based on miracles, however; it is based on certified knowledge and previous research on animals. Saying that the research did not benefit Baby Fae directly does not imply that it was unethical per se, but it does mean that such research should be subject to stringent standards.

- If the research did not benefit Baby Fae, did it involve more than minimal risk of harm? If so, was it a minor or a major increase? Clearly the surgery involved a major risk of harm. Not only was there the risk of immediate death, there was the certainty of physical pain and suffering from the surgery and deterioration of vital organs from the drugs used to suppress Baby Fae's immunological defenses. In addition to the risk of physical harm, the risk of emotional harm must be considered as well. Baby Fae spent her last days as a research object, not in the arms of a loving mother. In sum, the IRB at Loma Linda University did not have the right to approve the research on Baby Fae.

Conclusion

Because there was no hope of benefiting Baby Fae and because the risk of harm involved in the transplant procedure was a major increase over minimal harm, the baboon heart research proposal should have been submitted to a national panel of experts selected by the Secretary of Health and Human Services. Although research involving transplants from animals is not in itself unethical, it should be carried out only after the protocol, its scientific justification, and an analysis of risk and benefit have been evaluated and approved by a group of competent peers.

Note

1. *Research Involving Children* (Washington, D.C.: National Commission for Protection of Human Subjects of Biomedical and Behavioral Research, OS77-0004, 1977); *Federal Register* 48, no. 46 (March 8, 1983); "Additional Protection for Children Involved as Subjects of Research," *Federal Register,* 48, no. 46 (March 8, 1983).

Chapter 46 _____

Destroying One Life to Save Others

In April 1995 Baby K died, ending a two-and-a-half-year ethical and legal saga for this anencephalic child. She had received overly aggressive and inappropriate treatment at the behest of her mother despite the recommendations of the treating physicians. In stark contrast, in May 1995 the Council on Ethical and Judicial Affairs for the American Medical Association (AMA) advocated the removal of vital organs from live anencephalic children to provide organs for others in need.[1] In recommending such a policy, the Council reversed its previous opinion on the matter. The Council's recommendation represents the other extreme of dysfunctional ethical approaches to the care of individuals with this devastating congenital anomaly.

A middle ground allowing for the birth of an anencephalic infant followed by the provision of comfort care is most sound ethically. Yet an uncritical acceptance of faulty rationales supporting the extremes of killing the child or providing overly aggressive care hampers a movement toward the middle ground. Chapter 38 from this volume assessed the ethical propriety of the treatment of Baby K.[2] This chapter examines the defects in the arguments utilized by the AMA's Council to justify the use of live anencephalic infants as organ donors.

Theresa Ann Campo was born in Florida in 1996. In an effort to "make sense" of their child's anencephaly, her parents petitioned the courts to declare their daughter dead so that doctors could remove vital organs for transplantation. The Florida court rejected the parents' petition, affirming the current requirement for complete brain death before vital organ removal. Although efforts have surfaced periodically to amend the criteria for brain death to consist of cessation of neocortical or upper-brain activity, such a redefinition of death seems unlikely. An anencephalic infant clearly is human, albeit with impaired function, and has the ability to maintain homeostasis. One could hardly fathom burying such a child as though it were dead while the child still breathed of its own accord. Perhaps for that reason, the AMA Council's recent proposal eschews the journey down the semantic path of redefining death. The Council admits the neonate is alive and a person. The Council argues, however, that its life can be sacrificed for the sake of other goods. The Council defends its utilitarian position in a threefold manner. First, the Council appeals to the shortage of organs, which removal from anencephalic infants would ameliorate. Second, the Council indicates that anencephalic infants lack consciousness and normally have a limited life span. Third, the removal and transplantation of organs helps create meaning for parents in an otherwise "meaningless situation."

At first glance, the Council's opinion seems grossly utilitarian and even philosophically naive. Yet the Council recognized several countervailing positions and responded to them accordingly. To some of the objections, the Council provides adequate response. To the more substantial objections, however, the Council fails to provide convincing argumentation.

Discussion

The Council posits that some people object to removal of organs because the "false diagnosis of anencephaly may result in the death of neonates who could achieve consciousness." Although there are conditions that appear to be similar to anencephaly, the diagnosis is one of the most certain ones in medicine. Consequently, if one were to posit that removal of organs in and of itself is ethically acceptable, the level of certainty of diagnostic criteria seems sufficient to justify removal.

A second objection that the Council convincingly dismisses is that anencephalic donors should not be used because such "neonates would rarely be a source of organs for transplantation." Estimates of the number of children helped by donation range from less than 100 to thousands. The Council argues that if it were inherently acceptable to remove organs doing so would be worth the cost even if only a handful of children were saved. In this regard, the Council's response reflects a mainstream and accepted ethical approach to transplantation.

A third counterargument that the Council addresses is the objection that their policy would "undermine public confidence in the organ transplantation system," which already labors at times under the burden of mistrust. In fact, despite overwhelming approval for transplantation, many people currently refuse to donate because of fears that organs will be removed prior to death or that aggressive treatment will be withheld to hasten death for the sake of organ "harvestation." Undoubtedly, the Council's proposed practice would not contribute to greater trust in the system because of its crass utilitarian basis. As the Council explains, however, with proper safeguards and the utilization of pilot programs, one could empirically determine if the policy would have an adverse effect. Ethically, if one accepts the supposition that one may remove organs from a live infant, this argument reduces to an analysis that the Council asserts can only be resolved by empirical data rather than theoretical predictions.

The Council easily satisfies these "straw man" objections. One might therefore presume that the Council's answers to other arguments are equally satisfying. All of the foregoing arguments, however, rely on the presumption that the removal of vital organs from a living anencephalic (which results in the death of the infant) is not intrinsically wrong. Does the Council present a persuasive argument to substantiate this claim? The Council argues that the anencephalic infant has no interest in staying alive because the child will never obtain consciousness. Although this argument might justify the decision not to provide aggressive life support, the Council does not demonstrate logically why it supports the conceptual movement to act against the very life of the child. That is, the Council fails to show that the child has somehow lost its inherent right to life. Although the Council maintains that it repudiates the sentiment that the essential worth of a person depends on the quality of his or her life, its policy sends that very message. The Council seemingly chooses not to acknowledge that an ethical difference exists between allowing the anencephalic child to die and killing the child for its organs.

Perhaps aware of this weakness in its presentation, the Council backtracks and asserts that the right to life "is not an absolute value in the sense of overriding all other values. Rather, it must be balanced with other important social values, including, as in this case, the fundamental social value of saving lives." The Council reveals the essential utilitarian foundation of its argument. It implies that one can legitimate the direct killing of innocent human life if it somehow will benefit a greater number of lives. The Council provides no justification, however, for this ethical presumption; it merely assumes the veracity of its assertion. At a time when the public recoils from revelations of outrageous violations of patients' rights in government radiation studies and other medical experiments (all for the sake of others), the Council ironically proposes an even more heinous violation of a patient's right: the abrogation of the fundamental right to life upon which all other rights are predicated. This insidiously pragmatic approach to medical decision making, which bypasses the ethical nature of the means for the sake of the end, must be confronted. Even though the saving of other lives is important, it cannot be achieved at the expense of the lives of others. In sum, the Council fails to substantiate its vital premise and provide a convincing rationale to justify the direct killing of an innocent person for the sake of others.

A second objection for which the Council fails to provide a coherent response involves a "slippery slope" concern—namely, that other patients, such as those in persistent vegetative state (PVS) or extremely debilitated states, will be used as live donors. The Council counters that because such people have previously exhibited conscious behavior, they "have an interest in living" that distinguishes them from anencephalic infants. One can hardly imagine what those interests would be, however. Most people say "no" when asked if they would want to be kept alive if they were in a vegetative state. Cases such as those involving Nancy Cruzan and Christine Busalacchi substantiate that claim. Although one might be able to construct rare cases in which a PVS patient might want to be kept alive, one could posit the same to be true for an anencephalic infant who would be kept alive for the sake of parental need. The Council's argument is unconvincing because the policy moves out onto the slippery slope, with no logical barrier to prevent the progression down the slope. All of its essential arguments for the removal of organs from anencephalic infants apply equally to severely retarded or incapacitated persons, as well as PVS patients who seemingly lack an "interest in life."

Conclusion

The drive to obtain transplantable organs has led to outrageous statements with regard to anencephalic children. Some people have suggested that women who would normally abort their anencephalic children should be paid to carry the children to term so the organs can be "harvested." A surgeon at Loma Linda University stated that "it is ethically far more appropriate to use the organs of human infants who will die than those of animals who would otherwise have gone on living."[3] More insidious are proposals from respected organizations in health care that succumb to a utilitarian ethic. Even the American Academy of Pediatrics Committee on Bioethics, although currently opposed to adopting this new practice, indicates that it might be open to such a possibility under more favorable societal circumstances.[4]

Sound ethical theory acknowledges that certain actions are ethically unacceptable regardless of the benefit that might emerge. Sometimes we have to live with limitations. We will probably never have enough organs for transplants. Certain ethical standards cannot be compromised even for the sake of relieving suffering and death.

The need of parents to create meaning out the birth of an anencephalic child is profound and real. Consequently, we must help parents understand the goodness of the life they have created and help them with the grief process, just as one would with any child with a severe genetic deformity. As a society, however, we do parents a disservice by seeking to create meaning for them by killing their child. Although one need not provide aggressive life-sustaining interventions for the child with anencephaly, health care professionals must reverse the trend to abort anencephalics or the suggestion to kill them in an effort to "harvest" their organs.

Notes

1. Council on Ethical and Judicial Affairs, "The Use of Anencephalic Neonates as Organ Donors," *JAMA* 273 (1995): 1614–18.
2. See "Baby K: Is it Time to Take a Stand,?" chapter 38, pp. 138–41, this volume.
3. Steven Gundry, "Revisiting the Issues," *Update* 11 (July 1995): 6.
4. AAP Committee on Bioethics, "Infants with Anencephaly as Organ Sources: Ethical Considerations," *Pediatrics* 89 (1992): 1116–19.

Chapter 47 _____

Obtaining Organs from Non-Heart-Beating Cadavers

A physician gently informs Jane Smith's family that she will die of her condition regardless of life-support therapy. Because Jane had clearly stated that she didn't want to be "kept alive artificially" if there were no chance of recovery, the family asks the physician to remove the ventilator and allow their loved one to "die in peace." They ask, however, if she can be an organ donor because she had indicated so on her driver's license. Under controlled circumstances, the physician explains, it is possible for some patients to donate their kidneys (and sometimes the liver) after the ventilator is removed and death is pronounced. After much discussion, Jane's family signs the consent for donation and spends some final moments with her. Jane is then taken to the operating room, where the physician disconnects the ventilator. Soon Jane is unconscious, and she is draped for surgery. Her heartbeat becomes irregular; then the heart stops. After two minutes, death is pronounced, and the organ recovery team begins its work.

Jane Smith was treated in accordance with the University of Pittsburgh Medical Center's "Policy for the Management of Terminally Ill Patients Who May Become Organ Donors after Death."[1] Prior to the acceptance of brain-death criteria in the 1970s, non-heart-beating cadavers (NHBCs) served as a major source of transplantable kidneys, but their usefulness was generally limited by the prolonged interval between the declaration of death and the process of removing, cooling, and preserving organs. During this interval, organs endured warm ischemia, in which cell and tissue damage began and progressed—often to the point that the organs were irreparably damaged. In 1992, the University of Pittsburgh Medical Center circumvented this problem by procuring kidneys from persons who were pronounced dead shortly after a decision to forgo life-sustaining treatment. The potential contribution of NHBC organs is significant; data indicate that the use of such organs could increase the donor pool by 20–25 percent.[2]

Principles

Two important principles that provide the moral framework for organ procurement are that patients must be dead before their organs are taken, and the care of living patients must never be compromised in favor of potential organ recipients. One way to increase the organ supply without directly violating these principles is to take advantage of ambiguities in terminology for the current definition of death. Proponents of the Pittsburgh policy claim to accept the criteria for the determination of death as presented in the Uniform Definition of Death Act: either irreversible cessation of circulatory and respiratory functions or irreversible cessation of all functions of the entire brain, including the brain stem. How long must the heart have stopped beating before patients can justifiably be pronounced dead and their organs removed? When can we be confident that cardiopulmonary criteria have been met—that is, that the relevant functions have ceased irreversibly? Consider a woman who is found face down by the side of the road, apparently the victim of a single-car accident. Paramedics arrive within fifteen minutes of a call from a passing motorist. The patient is not breathing, has no pulse, and shows evidence of massive head injury. The emergency service personnel initiate (unsuccessfully) efforts at resuscitation and transport the patient to the local emergency department. The woman is declared dead by the emergency physician. When did she die? The time difference is small for deaths determined by cardiopulmonary criteria, but that short period is the precise issue in NHBC protocols.

Patients and their families deserve respect, dignity, and support as they face the reality of death. The interest in procuring organs must never adversely affect the care of the dying person and his or her family. When is it legitimate to undertake actions aimed at maintaining optimal functions of the organs to be retrieved? Clearly, the organ transplant team is free to do what is necessary to improve the utility of organs once the person is dead. In persons whose deaths are being closely monitored so that doctors can retrieve organs as quickly as possible, however, we must decide in a principled way which interventions are tolerable prior to the determination of death. The clearly living person who will become a donor must not be harmed, wronged, or killed. Choices often exist among possible plans of care that withdraw life-sustaining treatment and allow the patient to die. It seems legitimate to choose the plan that protects the organs best, provided that this choice does not cause the patient to suffer and that it reflects valid consent. Doing so will require being very careful not to create incentives to accelerate death improperly or allow any disrespectful treatment of the dying patient and family.

Discussion

A major criticism of the Pittsburgh protocol is that it might permit the removal of organs from patients who are not yet dead because it construes the concept of irreversibility too weakly. Under the Pittsburgh policy, doctors note the time that circulatory and respiratory functions cease and then wait two minutes for the documentation of one of three electrical dysfunctional rhythms of the heart (ventricular fibrillation, asystole, or electromechanical disassociation). At that point, the patient is declared dead. The protocol appears to demonstrate cessation of these functions, but is two minutes long enough to be confident that the cessation is *irreversible?* What about spontaneous auto-resuscitation? Theoretically, the health care team could intervene and successfully resuscitate the patient in that two-minute interval. Is the patient pronounced dead only because we have decided not to intervene with life-sustaining therapy?

Unfortunately, no one has studied a series of monitored patients being allowed to die in the same or similar conditions as the NHBC protocols propose. Ten of the twelve organizations reporting NHBC protocols in 1994 weaken the meaning of irreversibility even further by failing to specify a time limit between cessation of pulmonary functions and declaration of death. One of the protocols includes patients who are comatose, in a persistent vegetative state, or awake and alert. In this last scenario, a person with amyotrophic lateral sclerosis who had been living at home decided to end treatment and become an organ donor. He checked himself into the hospital, asked to be taken off life-support therapy, consented to donation, and eventually became an NHBC donor. An operating room nurse reported feeling that the procedure was "Kevorkian-like."

Protocols for NHBCs raise at least two concerns about family needs. First is a concern that families will be unable to say goodbye properly to their loved ones. The Pittsburgh protocol has been revised to allow families to say farewell at the moment of death in a private area near the operating room. Only three of the organizations in the 1994 study, however, gave families control over where their goodbyes would be said—the operating room, the intensive care unit, or a holding area outside the operating room. The second concern arises when the patient does not die as quickly as expected after the withdrawal of life support. Five organizations in the study had the experience of waiting in the operating room for periods of time ranging from 45 minutes to 10 hours before returning the patient to the unit. Several organizations have revised their protocols to include apnea testing prior to transporting the patient to the operating room.

Conclusion

Current NHBC protocols do not reliably and uniformly ensure that cardiopulmonary functions have ceased irreversibly before organ procurement begins. Much could be established by refraining from organ retrieval for a longer period of time following the cessation of cardiac and pulmonary functions. This longer observation period would also acknowledge the time in which a change in the plan of care might alter the outcome. In our zeal to save lives and allow people to give the "gift of life," we may fail to address the moral question that is posed by procuring organs from NHBCs: Are we manipulating the death of some persons to benefit others?

Notes

1. Stuart Younger et al., "Ethical, Psychosocial, and Public Policy Implications of Procuring Organs from Non-Heart-Beating Cadaver Donors," *JAMA* 269 (1993): 2769–74.
2. Bethany Spielman and Cynthia S. McCarthy, "Beyond Pittsburgh: Protocols for Controlled Non-Heart-Beating Cadaver Organ Recovery," *Kennedy Institute of Ethics Journal* 5 (1995): 323, 333.

Chapter 48 _____

Mandated Choice for Organ Donation

Organ transplantation is one of society's most dramatic medical success stories. Scores of lives are saved and dreams fulfilled. Yet every day, six persons will die while awaiting the procurement of suitable organs. In response to the dearth of organ donors, a policy of "mandated choice" has been suggested, by which individuals would be required to specify their organ donor status when they applied for driver's licenses, filed their tax returns, or obtained government identification cards. Proponents think the requirement would be a negligible intrusion, justified by the good that would come for those who need organ transplants and also because it amplifies the public's general support for the enterprise of organ transplantation.[1]

How society proceeds on this issue is more important than its conclusions. The problem of organ procurement is subtle and complex. To address it fruitfully, we need an open dialogue. Success will be marked by the emergence of shared civic ideals that unite clinicians, patients, and citizens on behalf of a common vision of organ transplantation and its value for human persons and communities.

Principles

There are at least three ways of conceiving organ donation. The first, simple philanthropy, may be the most popular. Simple philanthropy is distinguished from other forms of philanthropy by its emphasis on the originative will of the giver. According to this view, organ donation is an expression of the donor's spontaneous generosity. It is a gift in the supererogatory sense, neither required nor expected. There is no tie between donor and recipient, except in the sense that the former bestows a favor on the latter. Persons who hold that organ donation is an act of simple philanthropy object to conceiving it as an expected response or, worse, an obligation. They think social expectations for donation would infringe on human liberty by limiting the range of socially acceptable choices.

Social contract is a second conception. It begins with the recognition that most Americans approve of organ transplantation and expect it will be available if they need it. To expect such a service, according to this view, is to incur an obligation to support the enterprise of organ transplantation. Of course, if there are no donors, transplantation would be of no value to anyone. Hence, an implicit social contract holds that persons expecting to receive transplants must also resolve to be donors, should the occasion arise.

Persons subscribing to these first two conceptions tend to share a central belief that human fulfillment is engendered primarily by the satisfaction of personal preferences and desires. From such a perspective, establishing one's personhood is largely a matter of becoming independent. Independence, in turn, is a matter of extricating oneself from social influence so that one can determine one's destiny without interference. Although both positions concede that maximizing personal satisfaction will entail a degree of cooperation, neither views cooperation as a fundamental human value.

A third conception stands in contrast to the first two. In this view, donating an organ is an act of loyalty to the community. The moral relationship between individuals and communities embodied in this conception is too subtle and complex to be captured by the notion of contract; it is a covenant. Covenantal accounts of moral life begin with the observation that individuals are nurtured and sustained by communities. In return, the individual takes on a duty of fidelity to these communities. Expressions of covenantal fidelity cannot be prescribed entirely in advance. To a degree, they must be a creative undertaking, eclipsing mere obedience to a static code of behavior or execution of a contract. Such creativity is embodied in a life of loyalty to ideals that animate and define human communities.

From the perspective of covenant, freedom depends on the ability to serve a cause effectively and is contrasted to the paralysis of poor habits and worthless aims. The latter shortcomings are viewed as inevitable results of the paltry form of independence endorsed in the aforementioned conceptions. Human fulfillment based on covenant is a matter of living on behalf of shared ideals. The maximization of options or choices is not an unqualified good but is desirable insofar as it enriches the possibilities for such a life devoted to ideals.

According to the covenantal view, it is unlikely that organ donation would be explicitly required. Transplantation is not so central to our collective moral vision. On the other hand, the donation of an organ, on this view, is more than a spasm of generosity. Though the gift is not required, the loyalty that begets the giving *is* a requirement; it is part of a covenant between citizens and the community. Likewise, the relationship between donor and recipient is deep. Both are members of a community that endorses and potentiates the practice of organ transplantation. The gift is an authentic expression of the donor's loyalty to this community, an expression of personal identity. Moreover, it strengthens and enriches the covenant between recipient and community.

The covenantal model of organ donation is preferable to the other two models because it adequately reflects the evolutionary nature of human persons in human communities. Moral commitments cohere, on this model, with a primary insight of anthropology—that human persons are social beings, striving for communal ends.

Discussion

The current state of organ transplantation in the United States is something of a paradox. Healthy Americans consistently say they support it.

When in need of an organ, we favor the enterprise. Yet we generally do not donate our organs. The public philosophy seems to be that it is blessed to receive but not to give.

Mandated choice is a response to this discrepancy; it exhibits several positive features from a covenantal point of view. First, the policy is based on a presumption that most citizens will want to be donors. This presumption coheres with the viewpoint that good citizens are concerned for community welfare. Second, the policy preserves an element of choice, which is fundamental to loyalty. Presently, healthy persons have three options regarding organ donation: to choose donation (tentatively) in advance, to reject donation in advance, or to say nothing. Under mandated choice, only the first two options would remain for most persons. Having these two options may be more conducive to freedom in the covenantal sense (understood as maximizing the opportunities to serve a cause) than having all three. One could argue that the third option— saying nothing—functions mostly as a mechanism for allowing indecision or inertia to impede personal development and human progress.

Third, a policy of mandated choice would presumably spark public dialogue about organ transplantation and its role in human flourishing. Such dialogue is essential to forging the sort of community—and the sort of citizens—that can sustain a covenant. Fourth, decisions about organ donation are bound to be made more calmly and objectively in advance by the donor than at the time of death by the donor's grieving family. Such advance decision making would be promoted by mandated choice. Finally, the policy would probably increase the number of organ donors. This result would certainly be of benefit to organ recipients. Whether it would benefit the donors' families remains to be seen, although there is reason to think it would.

The considerations in favor of mandated choice may not be overwhelming. They are countered by several possible liabilities. Mandated choice is a procedural response to a problem that derives more from civic apathy than it does from unfairness or inefficiency. Bureaucratic solutions are not always the best remedy for apathy. There may be a less authoritarian way to stimulate public spirit. There are also concerns about the integrity of choices that would be made under the proposed policy. Would there be undue social pressure to decide in favor of donation, even when good reasons existed for declining? Would there be mechanisms for reversing a decision, once made? If so, how cumbersome would the process become, and how authoritative would the proposed advance directives be? Would family members still be called upon to authorize donations? Or would they be allowed to reverse donors' decisions only when they have good evidence that the deceased would do the same?

Conclusion

The poor rate of organ procurement in a society that approves of organ transplantation is disturbing. To a degree, this failure is a manifestation of weak communal bonds, resulting in mistrust, selfishness, and apathy. It also derives, however, from the current norm of thrusting decisions about organ donation on bereaved relatives. Mandated choice may be a partial remedy for both sources of failure. On the other hand, a policy of mandated choice may threaten the integrity of decisions about organ donation.

There should be a public dialogue on this matter. Organ donation and transplantation is best viewed as a community enterprise, enriching the lives of citizens as it beckons their support. Perhaps mandated choice could be part of a thriving community organ transplantation program. Perhaps other measures would be more equitable. The solution is not as clear as the means of initiating our inquiry. We should ask about the meaning of being a person in a community and explore the ways in which this meaning may be enriched through the enterprise of organ transplantation and organ donation.

Note

1. A. Spital, "Mandated Choice for Organ Donation: Time to Give it a Try," *Annals of Internal Medicine* 125 (1996): 66–69.

Part Six

Research

Chapter 49

Human Research Using Animals

In the nineteenth century, a movement to limit the use of animals in medical research began in England. Led by Frances Power Cobbe (1822–1904), the movement opposed animal vivisection—a term used to signify opposition to the use of animals, especially living animals, in any form of research. In response to the urging of several prominent citizens who supported the movement, the British Parliament in 1876 passed the Cruelty to Animals Act, which required the registration of places where experiments were performed on living animals, licensing of researchers, and permission for particular types of research. British antivivisectionists are still active and have had the regulations on animal research strengthened through subsequent laws in 1913 and 1965.

Not surprisingly, the movement spread to the United States, resulting in federal legislation that set limits and regulations on research with animals (1966). Significant limitations of animal research have also resulted from organized volunteer organizations such as the Institute for Study of Animal Problems (ISAP) and the Fund for the Replacement of Animals in Medical Experiments (FRAME). These more or less irenic organizations work openly in the public forum and promote their objectives through publicity and political action. More aggressive organizations such as People for Ethical Treatment of Animals (PETA) and the Animal Liberation Front (ALF) approve of direct attacks on research facilities. These groups seem to think that any action they perform to prevent research on animals is justified because they feel so strongly about it, and people start to listen if they destroy property.

Many people are not against using tissue from dead animals for research but seek to eliminate research on living animals. For others, putting animals to death to use them in research presents a problem. Proponents of this position argue that animal research is not necessary and that research projects using animals are ephemeral. For example, they assert that most experiments that use living animals are not for "medical" experiments but to test nonessential items such as cosmetics, shampoo, and food coloring. Finally, they maintain that computers could replace animals in most research projects. Researchers dispute this assertion, pointing out that in the past forty years, vaccine research—which has led to vaccines for polio, diphtheria, measles, mumps, whooping cough, and rubella—could never have been developed through computer models.

The Movement's Staying Power

In the face of obvious examples of the benefit of using animals in scientific research, what gives the antivivisectionist movement such staying power? Most of the anticruelty societies started in the nineteenth century have long since disbanded. Although the antivivisectionist movement has been less than popular in some areas of the United States, however, it never dies out. Indeed, it seems to have increased in numbers in the latter part of the twentieth century. There seem to be several reasons that attract people to the movement. Some people desire to protect animals from pain. As Jeremy Bentham stated in the eighteenth century, "The question is not can they reason, nor can they talk, but, can they suffer?" One response to this aphorism is to distinguish between pain and suffering. Although animals may experience pain, it is an instinctive reaction that does not connote true suffering—which requires the power of reflection in addition to sense cognition.

Some people adhere to the movement because they maintain that animals are not a different species from human beings and should not be considered at the disposal of human beings. Animals as well as humans, they maintain, should be protected from painful experiences because there is basically no difference between these two species of living beings. One spokesperson for this philosophy even maintains that there would be no difference between using retarded children instead of animals for research, even lethal research. Whether this theory—which equates animals and humans—is a cause or an effect of the antivivisectionist movement is not clear, although the movement existed long before this philosophical underpinning was developed. At any rate, until dogs and horses organize anticruelty societies in favor of their owners and masters, the argument equating animals and humans will remain in the realm of pure theory.

Another factor that enables the movement to survive is heavily publicized "abuses" in animal research. For example, in the early 1980s a center specializing in simian research was accused of keeping the apes and monkeys in filthy quarters. Also in the early 1980s, dogs were shot and wounded to enable military doctors to practice sewing gunshot wounds caused by a new type of ammunition. Both events led to an outcry by the well-organized animal rights societies and then by the general public. Court proceedings in response to the charges against the research scientists in the simian project show that an animal rights activist infiltrated the project. While other researchers were on vacation, he allowed conditions in the laboratory to deteriorate and then took pictures depicting "unsanitary conditions." Investigation of the wound-healing project revealed that the dogs were anesthetized before the research began and did not endure pain.

Although these theories and incidents give impetus to the movement, another influence seems to underly the longevity of the movement. This factor is seldom mentioned in studies in favor of or against animal research. This unmentioned factor is a feeling of mistrust that many people have for science, technology, and scientists. This mistrust develops into the attendant feeling that "all would be all right again" if we could only put science and technology back in the bottle. Because the general public apprehends scientists as engaged in occupations that are far removed from ordinary activities of daily life, they are prone to mistrust them and blame the shortcomings of technology on them. It is easy to depict scientists as using animals in a harmful manner because the ordinary person does not see the intimate connection between animal research and improved human health.

Toward a Solution

Considering the distance between scientists and the general population, it will be difficult to convince people of the value of animal research unless they realize the personal benefits that accrue from such protocols. With this challenge in mind, several physicians and scientists have organized a national group called the Incurable Ill for Animal Research (IIFAR) with the slogan "Lab animals save human lives and animal lives." The thrust of the organization's literature directly ties animal research to the future cure or alleviation of some of the fatal and debilitating diseases that afflict young and old in our country, such as cystic fibrosis, leukemia, and diabetes. Even with the formation of IIFAR, the antivivisectionists outspend by a wide margin those who see benefits to human life resulting from animal research.

The fundamental reason that justifies the use of animals in the quest for a better life for human beings is found in the relationship of humans to animals. Human beings demean themselves if they abuse animals. In the effort to prolong life, improve health, and foster the overall well-being of society, however, humans have a moral need and legal right to use animals, just as they have the need and right to use minerals and plants for the same purposes. Progress in culture and civilization are based on this common-sense teaching. Moreover, this principle is also the teaching of religions that seek to improve the human condition by recognizing that beings with spiritual faculties have the responsibility to act as stewards over other created beings.

Chapter 50

Use of Fetal Tissue in Research and Therapy

The ethical assessment of the use of fetal tissue for research or therapeutic purposes is deceptively easy at first glance. Regardless of the source of the tissue, the potential good to be done would seem to require that otherwise "wasted" fetal remains be put to some good use—whether for pure research or for the treatment of identified persons suffering from conditions such as Parkinson's disease, Alzheimer's disease, brain damage, or spinal cord injuries. The fact that some tissue might come from electively aborted fetuses may appear to be of little consequence in light of the hoped-for good to be achieved. Indeed, if one relies primarily on a utilitarian approach (i.e., an approach that argues that the good one seeks to accomplish can be pursued even if the means to that good are evil), one may be able to justify the use of fetal tissue from any available source.

Traditional medical ethics, however, has relied on principles other than utility in determining what is and is not ethically appropriate in the practice of medicine in the research and therapeutic settings. Thus, principles such as nonmaleficence and beneficence require that physicians refrain from harming persons; that they do not choose to do evil even if some good can be produced in the process; and that they always act in the best interests of persons.

Discussion

In applying these principles to the ethical assessment of the use of fetal tissue in research and therapy, we must address the source of the tissue. Once the source has been identified, the question to be answered is, "Is use of tissue from this source ethically justified?"

Generally, tissue for such purposes is available from either spontaneously aborted or electively aborted fetuses. In cases in which spontaneous abortion is the source, one would seem to be ethically justified in using the tissue for research or therapeutic purposes—providing, of course, that suitable respect is shown to the fetal remains and that appropriate consent is obtained from the parents.

The ethical evaluation of the use of tissue from elective or induced abortions recognizes that such abortion constitutes an evil in itself. This recognition requires that several questions be asked in making the ethical assessment. Does the use of electively aborted fetal tissue support the evil of abortion? Does the use of this tissue constitute complicity in the evil of abortion? Does the use of this tissue further the growth of the abortion industry to the extent that such use should be ethically proscribed?

Because of the potential for good from the use of this tissue, I would like to answer "no" to such questions—such use does not constitute ethically unacceptable cooperation in abortion. Caution must be exercised here, however, to ensure that the evil of abortion does not become institutionalized in our society because of an implicit justification it gains as we attempt to rationalize the use of electively aborted fetal tissue in the pursuit of some good(s).

Such a cautious approach must take account of the following factors. First, without the availability of fetal tissue there would be no possibility of benefit. Thus, any separation between research/therapeutic goals and abortion created by legal or other means is simply a fiction. Second, even if initially only fetal tissue from ethically acceptable sources is used, once the therapeutic possibilities become evident, the need and demand for wider availability of tissue will grow exponentially beyond what can be provided from spontaneous abortions. Third, the often painful decision to have an abortion could be mitigated by knowledge that some good could come from such a choice. The possibility of such relief could in turn lessen the reluctance to choose death over life when women face such options.

Recall the recent arguments made in favor of using anencephalic infants as organ donors—arguments made in favor of expanding the criteria for determining death in these newborns so that their organs would be more useful for others. The rationale for this approach (at least in part) was that the parents could feel that their baby's life or death had some meaning. What was understood as the source of that meaning, however? The baby's usefulness to another in need of a transplant.

Because medicine and its developing technologies are oriented to benefiting persons, the temptation will always exist to assess the appropriateness of methods for providing that benefit purely according to a utilitarian calculus, which always includes the ability to use evil as a means to achieve a good. Such an approach, however, threatens to supplant the fundamental ethical norms that inform traditional medical ethics (i.e., do no harm and benefit when able). Furthermore, utilitarian thinking tries to convince us that we may be justified in setting aside our commonly held views of what is morally appropriate given a potential benefit of great enough significance. That is the real danger here.

Conclusion

Unless great caution is exercised, we risk initiating a self-perpetuating process of justification whereby two things occur, both of which are equally unacceptable. First, the "evil" (i.e., individual abortions or the abortion industry in general) that we do or participate in, in the pursuit of the good (research/therapy), loses its significance for us as *evil*—or at least it takes on the identity of a "necessary evil" that we no longer find troubling. Second, the many "lesser" concerns (e.g., paying for fetal tissue to increase the supply, thereby increasing the number of abortions, or providing incentives for delaying abortion until the second or third trimesters to have more developed, more useful tissue/organs) become nonconcerns in light of the good that we propose to do.

The separation between the good that is hoped for and the evil used as a means to achieve that good must be complete and substantial. Until it is, the ethical appropriateness of using fetal tissue obtained from elective abortions (and perhaps even spontaneous abortions) will remain questionable.

Chapter 51 _____

Embryo Research: Ethical Issues

In 1994, a committee appointed to advise the National Institutes of Health (NIH) with regard to research on human embryos submitted its report.[1] The committee report includes the following conclusions:

1. Funding of research on human embryos with tax money is acceptable, but such research should be subject to strict guidelines.
2. The embryo merits significant respect as a developing form of human life, but this respect does not outweigh the potential value of embryo research.
3. Human embryos in the very early stages of development do not have the same moral status as infants and children.
4. Embryo research can make important contributions to a range of medical problems, including birth defects and certain types of cancer.
5. Human embryo research should be limited to about the first fourteen days—that is, until the embryo develops the "primal streak" that is the seminal formation of the central nervous system.

In sum, under recommendations of the NIH committee, researchers using federal funds would be allowed to fertilize human ova with human sperm with the sole purpose of submitting the resulting embryos to experimentations, intending to destroy them before they develop the "primal streak."

Principles

In the past, there have been several instances of research that violated the rights of human subjects. The Tuskeegee Project comes immediately to mind. As a result of the many abuses and aberrations in the field of research on human subjects, some ethical norms have been developed and affirmed by the scientific community. First, when making ethical judgments concerning research on human subjects, it is necessary to distinguish between therapeutic and nontherapeutic research. Therapeutic research aims at the well-being of the human subjects in the research project. Nontherapeutic research aims at providing new knowledge for the benefit of others and is not of benefit or value to the people in the research project. Second, regardless of whether the research is therapeutic or nontherapeutic, human persons must not be enrolled in research projects unless informed consent is obtained.

A third principle concerns the risk of serious harm that may result from research. If therapeutic research involves a risk of serious harm, the subjects or their proxies may accept the risk of serious harm as an unintended effect of the therapeutic endeavor. If the research is nontherapeutic, however, a person capable of giving informed consent may accept the risk, but a proxy cannot subject an incapacitated person to the risk of serious harm. The role of the proxy is to protect the ward from harm. To expose an incapacitated person to serious harm for the interest of science or society is to use that person as a thing and to demean or abuse his or her human worth.

Discussion

If we use the ethical norms for research agreed upon by the scientific community to evaluate the recommendations of the federal committee on embryo research, what conclusions may we draw? First, the question arises, Is the embryo a human subject? The NIH committee is ambivalent in this regard. Although the committee maintains that the human embryo at early stages of development does not have the same moral status as infants and children, the committee does not state anything more definite. One committee member declared, "An embryo merits significant respect as a developing form of human life, but their respect does not outweigh the potential benefits of embryo research." Apparently, the committee is willing to admit that the embryo is human with regard to its ontological being but not human insofar as protection from harm is concerned. At best, this concept is confusing. A being either is or is not human. Just as a woman cannot be "a little bit pregnant," an embryo cannot be a little bit human. If it is human, it deserves respect and protection simply because it is human.

The NIH committee seems to base the quality of being human on visual appearance (the primal streak), or self-awareness. Yet the constituent factor determining the presence of human life or personhood is not the physical appearance of a being, nor even self-awareness; it is the presence of a genetic code that enables the human entity to function in an integrated manner. The genetic code is disposed to a set of remarkable capacities. Contrary to the expressed thinking of the committee, from the earliest stage of development, the one- or two-celled zygote does have integrated activity. The reason it develops the primal streak and other physical characteristics, and eventually self-awareness, is because of its capacity for integrated human function in its earliest stages of life. Studying the same questions regarding the identity of the human embryo, a scientific commission in Australia stated, "No marker event (in the development of the embryo) carried such weight that different principles should apply to distinguish the fertilized ovum from that which all would agree is a human subject."[2] As a corollary of its study, the Australian commission rejected the distinction between an embryo and a pre-embryo.

The NIH committee seems intent to distinguish between a human being (physically developed, conscious, and self-aware) and developing human beings. No such distinction is logical. At all stages of human life, the human entity is "developing." There is no stage of physical or psychic development that allows others to say, "Now you are a human being because you will not develop any further." Being a developing entity is essential for human life. Different stages of development do not establish whether a human being is a person capable of possessing rights. True, some early stages of development may require that conscious and self-aware persons defend the rights of those who are not conscious or self-aware, but that is the nature of human community.

Is the type of embryo research envisioned by the committee therapeutic or nontherapeutic? Clearly it is nontherapeutic because the embryos will be destroyed within about fourteen days of their generation. Indeed, even though they could develop into human beings with self-awareness, the embryos are generated with the intention of killing them at a very early age. Given the proper protection and nourishment, these embryos of their own accord would develop into fully mature human beings. If the words of the NIH committee were not so tragic, they would be comical. The committee states, "An embryo meets significant respect as a developing form of human life," yet it is willing to subject the embryos to any and all forms of nontherapeutic research and then be destroyed. As one prominent ethicist remarked, "One wonders how the embryos would be treated if they did not merit significant respect as developing human life."

The unscientific and illogical ambiguities and equivocations of the NIH committee can only be explained by the desire for new knowledge. Theoretically, this research "can make important contributions to a whole range of medical problems, including birth defects, certain types of cancer, new methods of contraception, and in vitro fertilization." Clearly, the committee falls into the trap of pragmatism, as have other researchers in the past. According to the pragmatic credo, the end does justify the means; evil actions may be performed if the good seems to outweigh the evil. The heart of the problem seems to be that the panel doesn't realize the enormity of the evil that they are willing to tolerate to seek new knowledge. Once respect for individual human life is lost or devalued, all forms of degradation and exploitation follow logically in its wake.

Conclusion

In a move deemed politically motivated by the chair of the panel, President Clinton barred federal funding for research on embryos. Yet he allowed federal funding for research on embryos "left over" from IVF procedures. Congress has refused to allow funds to be alloted by the NIH for research on living fetuses.[3] Ethically speaking, the source of funding is irrelevant. The significant ethical issue is the respect due to human life at early stages of development.

Notes

1. "Federal Panel Urges U.S. to Drop Its Ban on Financing of Human Embryo Research," *New York Times* (September 27, 1994).
2. Senate Select Committee on the Human Embryo Experimentation Bill 1985, *Human Embryo Experimentation in Australia,* Australian Government Publishing Service, 1986.
3. S. S. Hall, "The Recycled Generation," *New York Times Magazine,* January 30, 2000.

Chapter 52 _____

Research in the Emergency Department

Paramedics bring a twenty-year-old man to the emergency department following a motorcycle accident. He has suffered severe trauma to the head. Physicians may have enough time to stop the bleeding before there is permanent damage to his brain. One of the potential treatments has not been tested in clinical trials. The patient is unconscious, and no family member is available to approve the attempt to save his life. This situation is not uncommon. In emergencies, physicians frequently make split-second decisions about which therapies offer the best chance for survival. Trauma victims often owe their lives to treatments given while they were unconscious. To foster access to potentially lifesaving treatment, the Food and Drug Administration (FDA) approved regulations in October 1996 to ease informed consent requirements for experimental treatment in emergency situations if a research protocol has already been approved.[1]

The new FDA rule represents the first substantive change in the informed consent ethic since the enactment of the Nuremberg Code more than fifty years ago. The agency claims that much of the standard medical therapy used in acute clinical care has not been adequately evaluated through clinical trials. FDA regulators expect the informed consent waiver to improve the efficacy and safety of treatments that currently have poor clinical outcomes. This unprecedented move presents an opportunity to consider the ethical norms of informed consent and research. Does the potential benefit of treatment that is untested in formal clinical trials outweigh the general requirement to obtain consent? How do we balance the need for research in emergency room treatments with careful attention to the welfare of severely injured patients?

Principles

Informed consent is at the heart of ethical research. It is rooted in respect for persons—a principle that regards individuals as autonomous agents capable of deliberation about personal goals and of acting under the direction of such deliberation. International ethical codes and human rights laws accept informed consent as a universal expression of respect that incorporates at least two basic convictions: first, that individuals are autonomous agents, and second, that persons with diminished capacity deserve protection. Respect for persons thus divides into two separate moral requirements: the requirement to acknowledge autonomy and the requirement to safeguard those who are incapable of making autonomous decisions. The consent process is ideally collaborative in nature because physicians and patients have essential information regarding the physical, emotional, social, and spiritual needs of patients. The ultimate responsibility for decision making rests with patients, or their surrogates, if patients are incapable of making decisions.

The ethical responsibility to work for the overall benefit of patients presents particular challenges to physicians in clinical research. When science takes humans as subjects, tensions arise between two values basic to Western society: freedom of scientific inquiry and protection of individual inviolability. Research should contribute to generalizable knowledge for the good of people in the future and protect subjects from the risk of unnecessary harm. Although we can never eliminate risks, we can reduce them to only those risks necessary to achieve the research outcomes. Thus, ethical research must satisfy several requirements: The knowledge sought must be important and obtainable by no other means; appropriate experimentation must be done on animals or cadavers first; the probable risks of research must be proportionate to the potential benefits; selection of subjects and distribution of risks should be equitable; subjects must be free to withdraw from the research at any time without penalty. It is appropriate to ask human subjects for consent to participate in research only after these conditions are met.

We must distinguish between research on the one hand and the practice of accepted therapy on the other. Practice involves interventions that are designed solely to enhance the well-being of an individual patient and have a reasonable expectation of success. Research designates an activity that is designed to test a hypothesis, draw conclusions, and develop or contribute to generalizable knowledge. When a clinician departs in a significant way from standard or accepted practice, the innovation does not necessarily constitute research if there is no formal structure in place to evaluate outcomes. Unless there is a formal protocol to guide the project and its results, in essence it is simply an experimental treatment.

Discussion

An exception to fully informed consent already exists in emergencies when patients may lack decision-making capacity, no surrogate is available, and the need for treatment is urgent. For example, paramedics would presume consent for emergency treatment if they found a severely injured unconscious person at the scene of an accident. It seems reasonable to extend this exception to approved clinical trials in life-threatening situations. Critics of the FDA regulation argue that the potential for abuse of subjects will always be unacceptably high without strict requirements for informed consent. They contend that it is unethical for patients who cannot consent to receive experimental treatment.

We can examine the adequacy of the safeguards in the FDA rule in protecting subjects with diminished capacity. First, the FDA requires that the extent of protection for patients with diminished capacity be proportionate to the risks and likely benefits. To this end, the local institutional review board (IRB) must confirm that results from animal and other studies support the potential of providing benefit to individual patients directly. Second, the protocol must include procedures to inform surrogates immediately of the patient's inclusion in the research program. In addition, the surrogate must be informed about the details of the research and the option to withdraw from the protocol. Finally, the FDA requires consultation with representatives of the communities from which subjects will be drawn before initiation of any clinical trials. In these open meetings, researchers must describe the design, risks, and benefits of the proposed research. Some minority and economically disadvantaged communities that have higher percentages of refusals for participation in research argue that justice requires such public disclosure. If those communities object to the protocols, the researchers should give serious consideration to doing the research elsewhere.

Conclusion

Well-designed, previously approved clinical trials that allow access to potentially lifesaving therapies could suspend the obligation to obtain informed consent until a surrogate can be located. Local communities should be informed about the proposed research. IRBs must ensure that the research has the potential to benefit individual patients directly and that decisions to enroll specific patients in the research are appropriate. We must not send the message to the research community or the public that it is more important for clinical trials to continue than it is to protect individual autonomy. If we condone research that violates human rights, the public may see researchers and pharmaceutical companies as the worst sort of opportunists who experiment on comatose patients without consent.

We should make radically new departures from practice the object of formal research at an early stage. In that way, we can determine whether they are safe and efficacious. If there is any element of research in the therapy offered by physicians in the emergency department, the IRB should review it for the protection of the human subjects involved. A structured clinical trial will evaluate the therapy in a more systematic way. The FDA regulation could facilitate research in this patient population and provide necessary safeguards to ensure responsible and ethical research. Ultimately, such research could improve the availability of products proven efficacious to individuals in life-threatening situations.

Note

1. *61 Federal Register* (October 2, 1996): 471–531.

Part Seven

Suicide and Physician-Assisted Suicide

Chapter 53

Suicide: A Rational Choice?

In discussing ethical issues surrounding suicide, our main question is not, "Should people who commit suicide be criticized?" Experience and intuition demonstrate that most persons who take their own lives do so because they are emotionally disturbed and act compulsively. Thus, their freedom of choice is greatly restricted or nonexistent. Too many of us know dear friends or family members whose suicidal deaths demonstrate this lack of psychological freedom. Indeed, many experts in suicidology today seem to take for granted that all suicides are compulsive and irrational. Our question in this chapter, then, concerns the contemporary tendency to present suicide as a "rational choice"—that is, to present it as the best manner to die in some circumstances.

Principles

Among the ancient Greeks and Romans, suicide was both condemned and defended, as it also was in Eastern cultures. The Epicureans, who considered pleasure and peace of mind the highest good, argued that it was better to kill oneself than endure life if it had become more painful than pleasurable or peaceful. The Stoics, who believed that rigid self-control was the highest good, argued that it was permissible to kill oneself if suffering or torture might force one to lose self-control. Dualists taught that the soul, which is the real person, is burdened by the body in this life; hence, suicide might be justified as a laying down of this burden. Even today, some people believe it ethical to choose suicide for the sake of honor. Recently, some Irish and Vietnamese protesters chose suicide by self-starvation and self-immolation to protest injustice and oppression.

The monotheistic religions of Judaism, Christianity, and Islam have always opposed suicide because they regard life as God's gift, which people must use not as owners but as faithful stewards. Consequently, we cannot escape accounting to God for our stewardship of this one life given on earth, nor can we reject the body, which will always be part of us. This view was anticipated by Plato, who argued that suicide is a rejection of the responsibility to self, to the community of which one is a part, and to God who gave life. In a different way, Immanuel Kant argued that suicide is the greatest of crimes because it is a person's rejection of morality itself because a human being must be his or her own moral lawgiver. Committing suicide means treating oneself as a thing (means) rather than as a person (an end in oneself). In sum, in theological and philosophical reasoning, suicide has been considered for centuries as an unethical act, even though responsibility was seldom imputed to the unfortunate persons who performed the action.

Discussion

Today, however, this classic stand expressed in the monotheistic religions is being called into question. In the United States and England, societies promote suicide as an ethical action, a "rational" alternative to life, especially if a person is beset by depression, loneliness, severe infirmity, or serious suffering. Usually the reasons put forward for approving suicide as an ethical choice are that people should have the right to be autonomous and to control their own destiny or that people should not have to suffer pain, loneliness, or degradation at the time of death. Although these are the professed reasons for the modern reexamination of the traditional stance, noted psychiatrist and suicidologist David Peretz sees a more subtle cause for this change of thought:

> Under the unprecedented stress of recent decades, denial mechanisms are breaking down and we have become increasingly vulnerable to the threats of intensely painful feelings of anxiety, fear, panic, rage, guilt, shame, grief, longing and helplessness. In order to avoid being overwhelmed, we seek new ways to adapt. . . . I believe that the growing concern with a good death, death with dignity and the right-to-die reflect this search. . . . If our deepest known fear is of being destroyed, and we cannot deal with that fear, we take refuge in planning death and rational suicide. We find

comfort in the illusion, "It will not be done to me. . . . I will do it myself.[1]

Peretz feels that this motivation is dangerous because it fosters the harmful illusion of personal omnipotence.

Two other unrealistic and therefore unethical elements are involved in rational suicide. First, the call for rational suicide is based on the notion that personal autonomy or independence is the goal of human life. Rational suicide advocates argue that if one cannot be autonomous or independent, life is not worth living. This argument is simply one more expression of radical individualism—a philosophy that weakens human community and places little value on social justice. Experience and wisdom demonstrate, however, that interdependence, not independence, is the goal of human life. To admit that one is weak and needs help is not a denial or a perversion of one's humanity. Instead, accepting help is a means to fulfill one's humanity. The weak and suffering offer an opportunity to others to fulfill their humanity by responding with care and kindness. The perfectly autonomous person would not need other people; can one imagine a more boring and self-centered individual?

A second unethical element in rational suicide is that it mythologizes the act of self-destruction. To mythologize something is to give it powers it does not possess. Rational suicide advocates present self-destruction as a problem-free solution to the very serious human problems of physical suffering, loneliness, severe depression, or infirm old age. We do not eliminate human problems by eliminating human beings, however. We eliminate or alleviate human problems through compassion, care, and loving concern. The problems that rational suicide would pretend to eliminate are often problems with which individuals learn to live through the help of caring relatives or friends.

Conclusion

The present-day emphasis on the "right to die" and "death with dignity" may blind us to the right to life of the weak, infirm, and aged. The cost of combating the human problems of loneliness, infirmity, and depression is not self-destruction; it is the development of a compassionate, caring, and generous community. Although such caring is not simple, it is a development rather than a perversion of our humanity.

Note

1. David Peretz, "The Illusion of Rational Suicide," *Hastings Center Report* 11 (1981): 40–42.

Chapter 54
The Myth of "Managed Death"

A few years ago voters in the state of Washington defeated an initiative that proposed to legalize active euthanasia and assisted suicide. Had the initiative passed, conscious and competent patients in terminal conditions who had less than six months to live could have requested and received "aid in dying" from their physicians. Proponents of active euthanasia and assisted suicide argued that medicalized killing is the final and appropriate caring intervention of the physician in the life of a patient. Moreover, this "aid in dying" allows patients and physicians to manage death, thereby "taking responsibility for our technology, by assuring people who are its subjects that they will not be crucified on a cross of steel operating tables, shunts and tubes."

Many opponents of the initiative argued that concerns about the sanctity and inviolability of human life were enough to demonstrate the wrongness of the proposals. Others argued that even if there may be some justification for responding to the request for assistance when the competent patient asks to be killed, legalizing such practices would place society and the medical profession at the peak of the well-worn "slippery slope." In no time, they argued, we would be euthanizing the incompetent and the elderly in an attempt to bring health care costs under control—or for some other, less noble, reason. Still others maintained that society should neither ask nor allow its physicians to do things that might undermine the trust we place in them by permitting them to engage in actions that are inconsistent with the identity of "physician as healer."

The debate raised by proposals to legalize euthanasia and assisted suicide too often takes place in a context of confusion. This confusion results in a lack of clarity about what euthanasia and assisted suicide mean and involve.

For example, many people incorrectly include under the broad category of "euthanasia" not only killing upon request but also removal of useless or excessively burdensome life support, as well as the provision of adequate pain relief that may hasten death as a secondary effect. In addition, because the discussion of euthanasia and assisted suicide often begins with claims about a right to die, many people conclude that the ethical issue is simply one of responding to the requests of autonomous patients. Framed this way, the issues are interpreted almost exclusively in terms of questions about control. How can the suffering or dying patient maintain some semblance of control in what many people argue is a situation that inevitably "robs the person of dignity?" By concluding that "I will do it to myself, before it is done to me."

Clarifying the Issues

To assess ethically proposals for legalized euthanasia and assisted suicide, we must define terms and clarify the confusions noted above. Accordingly, *suicide* is a voluntary act by which one intends and causes one's own death. Suicide can be accomplished by acts of commission (e.g., shooting oneself) or by acts of omission (e.g., starving oneself to death). What is common to both is the introduction of a cause of death. *Assisted suicide* implies that the person cannot accomplish the intention or action to bring death about alone. Assistance in the suicide of another person can be accomplished by acts of commission (e.g., prescribing a lethal dose of medication and instructing the person in its use). Assistance also can be rendered in a more passive way through persuasion and encouragement. In either case, the person who contributes to the death-dealing effort shares in the intention to bring death about through the introduction of a causative agent.

Euthanasia, whether active or passive, is an act or an omission that of itself or by intention causes death. Euthanasia can be accomplished by actively introducing a cause of death not already present (e.g., by lethal injection) or by failing to circumvent the deadly effects of a cause already present when there is a duty to do so (e.g., withholding antibiotics to treat pneumonia in a child with Down's syndrome *because* of the Down's syndrome).

Assisted suicide and euthanasia are clearly distinct from the ethical decision to withhold or withdraw ineffective or seriously burdensome life-prolonging therapies. When life is threatened by a condition internal to the person—that is, by a fatal pathology—the cause of death is already present. If life-prolonging therapies can offer the patient no benefit, their removal is not a decision to kill the patient. Instead, it is a decision to forgo interventions that are ineffective or impose serious burden. Although in such circumstances death may be welcomed as a release from suffering, it is neither intended nor caused as a means to overcome suffering.

Finally, proposals to respond to suffering by offering a "managed death" simply mean that the one who suffers is eliminated. Such a response neither ensures control over the dying process nor enhances the dignity of the one who suffers. In The Netherlands, physicians are protected from criminal prosecution if they respond to the requests of patients for assisted death, providing they meet several criteria. One such criterion is that there must be suffering that the person describes as intolerable. Many Dutch physicians claim that most, if not all, physical pain can be controlled by the judicious use of medication. Thus, the kind of suffering that leads most terminally ill patients in The Netherlands to request active euthanasia is emotional or psychological suffering—that is, suffering that is dependent on subjective elements that often cannot be addressed effectively.

Since Elizabeth Kubler-Ross did her groundbreaking work with the dying, however, we have learned a good deal about the content of the psychological suffering that terminally ill persons experience. They suffer from fear of the unknown that naturally accompanies the dying process. They suffer from the fear of becoming a burden to their families and loved ones as they become less able to care for themselves. They suffer from the fear of being isolated from others by an experience that can only be understood fully by the one having it. And they suffer from fear of being abandoned by family, friends, and caregivers. Certainly, these forms of suffering pose significant challenges to caregivers. Yet the hospice experience has taught us that the willingness to accompany the dying person on the journey toward death goes a long way toward addressing these deeper levels of suffering. Hospice has also shown us that physical suffering can be managed by a commitment to provide adequate and appropriate pain relief. Finally, hospice programs reassure patients and families that although sophisticated technologies that can only prolong the dying process will not be used in the final days of life, other forms of appropriate care will be provided, and the dying person will not be abandoned.

Conclusion

The question to be answered, then, is this: Is "aid in dying" or managed death an ethically appropriate response to the needs and suffering of terminally ill persons? Although some people may disagree, the common moral vision in Western society consistently has answered "no" to this question.

The basis for this response is the conviction that certain kinds of intentions, and the actions to accomplish them, are beyond the authority of human agents. The killing of innocent human beings by one's own volition not only inflicts harm on the one killed but harms society as well. Killing actions do nothing to address the realities that cause suffering for terminally ill persons. Legalizing such actions only ensures that less effort will be expended by caregivers and others in the future in attempting to respond appropriately to the needs of persons who are dying.

Chapter 55

Kevorkian's Dilemma: Are We Owners or Stewards of Human Life?

Dr. Jack Kevorkian strikes again. Kevorkian, the retired pathologist who designed a death machine, has assisted at least nineteen people to commit suicide. His actions have evoked criticism and even outrage from people in the medical, legal, and ethical professions, as well as from leaders of religious communities. But, many people seem to agree with him.

There is certain logic in Kevorkian's efforts to assist people to commit suicide. Anyone who subscribes to the interpretation of autonomy favored by some legal decisions in the United States will find some meaning in the Kevorkian death machine. This legal interpretation is founded in the oft-quoted dictum of former Supreme Court Justice Benjamin Cardozo, "Every human being of adult years and sound mind has the right to determine what will be done with his own body."

Cardozo's dictum is rooted in Enlightenment thinking and is best expressed in the writings of John Locke, who regarded the state merely as a vehicle for protecting individual rights. Not irrationally, Justice Cardozo's dictum has been interpreted by many legal experts and ethicists to indicate that human beings have absolute dominion over their bodies and thus their lives in the same way that they would have dominion over a piece of property.

Just as persons may use, sell, or even destroy a car or a suit of clothing as it pleases them, they have the same power over their bodies and thus their lives. According to this view of human life and freedom, suicide becomes a "right," and if a person needs assistance in committing suicide, then there is a "right" to the assistance that is needed. Although Cardozo's words originally were used to demonstrate the need for informed consent before invasive medical procedures were performed, it does not take much imagination to use them in defense of suicide and assisted suicide.

Opposed to this concept of absolute dominion over body and life is a concept that envisions persons as stewards or caretakers of their bodies and their lives. Stewardship recognizes the power of the person to make free decisions designed to achieve the goods and goals of life. Stewardship also posits, however, that there are goods and goals of life that are innate. Indeed, the most fundamental and important goods and goals of life are innate.

The stewardship concept of the human person assumes that our drive toward worshiping God; respecting life as a gift; honoring one's parents; and striving for happiness, self-esteem, friendship, creativity, truth, and longevity arise from our very nature. The U.S. Constitution codified these innate goods and goals as "life, liberty, and the pursuit of happiness." These and other significant objectives toward which we direct our affections and actions result from the fact that we are not free to choose or reject the basic goals of life. Accordingly, in the stewardship view of the human person, killing oneself has always been considered a harmful action because it makes it impossible to strive for the basic goods of life.

The concept of stewardship is founded not merely in religious teaching or in mythology. It proceeds from an understanding that each person has innate goods and goals for which he or she strives and that some actions are helpful in achieving these goals, whereas other actions are detrimental insofar as achieving these goals are concerned. Killing innocent people, for example, has been rejected as incompatible with the goods and goals of life. Nourishing and caring for infants has always been considered an act that fulfills the goods and goals of life. This view of the person, his or her moral responsibilities, and the rejection of suicide and assisted suicide has been accepted in Western society much more than the opposite attitude. If the view of a person as owner of his or her body and life is so opposed to the view that has been traditional in Western society, why do so many people support the efforts of Dr. Kevorkian, and why is there a waiting list for the use of his suicide device? Why did Cardozo's dictum take so long to surface as a justification for suicide and assisted suicide? Why is there a tendency today to accept suicide and physician-assisted suicide, when accepting these actions would have been unthinkable twenty years ago?

Although several factors in our society contribute to the acceptance of suicide and assisted suicide as legal and ethical options, the following factors seem most significant.

First, our society is characterized by the philosophy of individualism as opposed to communitarianism. Individualism leads us to think that our well-being and self-worth depend on our ability "to take care of ourselves." Individualism not only teaches us to depend on our own resources exclusively; it tends to make us think that we are bad people or social failures if we must depend on others. How often do we hear people say, "I don't want to be a burden to others"? Faced with a choice between "being a burden" or suicide, some people under the influence of individualism will opt for suicide. Often, many people in a person's family or social unit may be capable of rendering compassionate help, but the help is not accepted because the individualistic person, even when suffering, habitually rejects the help of others. Expecting an aging or chronically ill person to be independent and "not a burden" is as foolish as expecting a newborn baby to be independent and "not a burden." Sometimes, acknowledging dependence is a very natural and beneficial recognition.

Second, self-worth in our society is assumed to depend on the individual's ability to contribute to economic productivity. In a more communitarian view of the person, the worth and value of the individual are based on his or her human nature. With this view of people who can no longer contribute actively as economic factors in society, depression and despair are avoided through compassionate care of suffering people.

Finally, many people are disposed to choose suicide because they fear losing control of their lives as death approaches; thus, they are tempted to choose suicide as a means of exercising control over their lives. Specifically, people who envision death, especially those in pain, fear that their lives will be prolonged through medical therapy that is not truly beneficial. Moreover, they fear that their pain will not be controlled. Although both of these fears have some basis in reality, efforts to overcome both aberrations of medical practice are being addressed in medical schools and residency programs. Because of American medicine's unquestioning acceptance of technology, the tendency to overtreat patients as death approaches will be more difficult to overcome than the undertreatment of pain. The acceptance granted to Kevorkian's plan and the tendency of some physicians to help their patients commit suicide are symptoms of a profession that is not able to handle death in an ennobling and supportive manner.

Depending on the way in which one views human responsibility, one will accept or reject suicide and physician-assisted suicide as ethical choices. Are we owners or stewards of human life? If we are owners of human life, then humans set their own standards for right and wrong behavior. With this exaggerated view of human dominion, however, ethics becomes a word game, society a jungle, and each person a ruler of his or her own world—as Niechtze predicted. On the other hand, if we are stewards of body and life, our fulfillment consists in striving for the goods and goals of life, the most important of which are innate.

Chapter 56

Physician-Assisted Suicide

In a 1994 issue of the *New England Journal of Medicine,* a group of physicians, assisted by a lawyer and a philosopher, defend physician-assisted suicide.[1] Realizing that physician-assisted suicide is "outside standard medical practice" and that it could lead to the abuse of vulnerable patients and the degradation of the medical profession, the authors devote most of their attention to developing a complicated process of regulating the manner in which requests for assisted suicide are evaluated and monitored.

Principles

Before we address the ethical arguments in the article itself, let us be clear about the subject matter. Usually, physician-assisted suicide implies that a physician provides the material needed for the suicide to be carried out by the patient. For example, the physician may supply lethal doses of medication that enable a person to kill herself or himself. Although the physician does not cooperate physically in the suicide of the patient, the physician cooperates morally in the suicide by approving the act of suicide, even if reluctantly. Thus, physician-assisted suicide is a moral participation in the killing of an innocent person. In the article under consideration, however, the authors also approve active euthanasia on the part of the physician—that is, the physical termination of a patient's life if the patient requests it. The extension of assisted suicide (a less proximate and direct involvement in the death of a patient) to euthanasia (direct and intended killing) is logical: If moral cooperation in an assisted suicide can be justified, why not the direct act of killing? According to the authors, the reasons that justify the act of cooperating in suicide or killing a person without the person's physical participation in the act (active euthanasia) are the patient's right of self-determination and the physician's responsibility to relieve pain.

Finally, physician-assisted suicide is not to be confused with the aggressive use of medication to relieve pain, which indirectly and beyond the intention of patient and physician might hasten the death of a suffering person. This form of aggressive comfort care for dying patients, as the authors acknowledge, is ethically acceptable and not under discussion in the article.

Discussion

As is often the case, the article presupposes some vital facts or ethical theories and then draws conclusions without examining the presuppositions on which the conclusions are based. The remaining part of this analysis considers and evaluates three of these presuppositions.

Presupposition 1

People suffering from intolerable pain that cannot be alleviated through comfort care are capable of making voluntary decisions. In fact, a desire to commit suicide, even when one suffers from pain or has a terminal illness, is interpreted by experts as an expression of depression. How can a person make a voluntary request to kill oneself, or be killed by a physician, if he of she is in a depressed condition? Recently, the New York Task Force on Life and the Law considered the feasibility of legislation to approve physician-assisted suicide but rejected the proposal, offering a much more realistic response. It stated, "For purposes of public debate, one can posit 'ideal' cases in which all the recommended safeguards would be satisfied: Patients would be screened for depression and offered treatment, effective pain medication would be available, and all patients would have a supportive, committed family and doctor. Yet the reality of existing medical practice in doctors' offices and hospitals across the state generally cannot match these expectations, however many guidelines or safeguards might be framed. These realities render legislation to legalize assisted suicide and euthanasia vulnerable to error and abuse for all members of society, not only for those who are disadvantaged." In sum, the presupposition that dying patients are capable of making voluntary decisions concerning suicide or direct killing—that is, decisions that are free from moral coercion—is simply unrealistic.

Presupposition 2

Physicians are the proper and exclusive agents for helping people cope with pain and approaching death. Thus, when physicians are unable to alleviate pain, they have failed in their profession. The authors presuppose that in the presence of pain that cannot be alleviated through medical care, the only alternative is patient- or physician-inflicted death. Even if we admit for the moment that pain cannot be controlled—an admission with which many pain specialists are not willing to agree[2]—assistance to cope with pain is available from many people besides those in the medical profession. Many people live with pain and in the face of death gain strength from their family and friends. Pain is not only a physiological phenomenon; it may occur at any level of human function: physiological, psychological, or psychic. A holistic evaluation of a dying person's situation requires a distinction between pain and suffering—a distinction not made in the article under study. Often, people can bear pain if loved ones share their suffering. The assumption that only members of the medical profession are responsible for and capable of helping people cope with pain and imminent death is short-sighted. In addition, it bespeaks a latent paternalism that the authors of this article would loudly denounce in other circumstances.

The notion that the inability to relieve suffering constitutes failure on the part of the physician is also misguided. Who does not know that death is inevitable? Who does not acknowledge that there will be pain and suffering in life that cannot always be overcome? Severe suffering and death are just as much a part of nature as birth and life. The nobility of the human person is found in coping with suffering if it cannot be overcome, not in surrendering to it through despair and suicide. Do we value people who give up in the face of adversity?

Presupposition 3

The intention of the agent is the only source of ethical decision making. Thus, an act that is unethical in itself may become ethical by reason of the good intention of the person performing the action. Thus, lying or cheating on an exam, which are wrong in themselves, will be defended as morally good if the person who performs them may suffer the harm of embarrassment or failure if he or she doesn't lie or cheat. The desire to judge the morality of human acts by the intention of the agent and to ignore the moral object of the action occurs throughout history. In generic terms, it is known as relativism. Elizabeth Anscombe, the great British philosopher, explained the distinction between the moral object and the intention of the agent in the following manner: "Whatever ulterior intentions you may or may not have, the question first arises: What intention is inherent in the action you are actually performing? What are you here and now doing on purpose? Whatever your ulterior aims, what one is here and now doing on purpose, precisely is called the object of the moral act."[3]

Although the intention of the agent is one source of morality, the primary determinant of ethical or moral identity is the moral object: "What you are here and now doing on purpose." The primary determinant of morality, the moral object, cannot be finessed or overridden by the intention of the agent. If that were possible, there would be no such thing as an unethical or immoral human act because people always have (what seems to them at least) a good intention for their actions. Some actions are always wrong, no matter what the intention of the agent. Would it ever be ethically acceptable to sell children into slavery, even if the intention of the agent were to provide a better life for the children?

Clearly, the authors of this article consider physician-assisted suicide generally to be unethical because they allow it only as a last resort. Moreover, they admit that any treatment whose purpose is to cause death "lies outside standard medical practice." The elaborate process calling for palliative care consultants and palliative care committees to assure that physician-assisted suicide is carefully controlled also indicates that suicide and euthanasia are immoral by reason of the moral object. When the authors maintain that to eliminate pain or to respect the patient's right to self determination a physician may assist a suicide or perform euthanasia, they are simply saying that one may do serious evil to achieve good.

Conclusion

The authors of the article maintain that through assisted suicide or euthanasia they seek to "relieve symptoms, and enhance the quality and meaning of life." This is double talk. As Leon Kass stated, "We cannot serve the patient's good by deliberately eliminating the patient."[4]

Notes

1. F. G. Miller et al., "Regulating Physician Assisted Death," *NEJM* 331:2 July 14, 1994: 119–124.
2. A. Jacox et al., "New Clinical Practice Guidelines for the Management of Pain in Patients with Cancer," *NEJM* 330 (March 3, 1994): 651–655.
3. Elizabeth Anscombe, *Ethics, Religion and Politics,* vol. III (Oxford, U.K.: Blackwell, 1981), 86.
4. Leon Kass, "Is There a Right? to Die," *Hastings Report* 23:11 (Jan–Feb 1993): 34–43.

*Chapter 57*_____

Suffering and the Debate Over Assisted Suicide and Euthanasia

The goal of ethics and ethical analysis is to promote and sustain the moral community of concern wherein life is possible and can flourish. Persons interested in ethics, therefore, must be distressed by any threat posed to the integrity of the moral community. Threatening the bonds of the community risks not only the well-being of individual persons in the present moment, it imperils all persons now and in the future by undermining the possibility of creating community.

The Protestant ethicist Paul Ramsey began his classic work *The Patient as Person* with an insight pertinent to this discussion. "We are born within covenants of life with life. By nature, choice or need we live with our fellow man in roles or relations. Therefore we must ask, What is the meaning of the faithfulness of one human being to another in every one of these relations? This is the ethical question."[1]

We live in a society that frequently scoffs at any claims about the need for fidelity in human relationships because fidelity implies not only individual rights but responsibilities as well. Within this environment, threats to the well-being of the community often are underestimated. A threat of significant proportions materialized on November 8, 1994. On that day, Oregon became the first state and the United States the first nation to make it legal for a physician to assist a person to commit suicide. The Oregon law allows a terminally ill adult who is capable of making an informed decision to make a written request for medication to end life in a "humane and dignified manner." Passage of this bill represents another misguided attempt to define the parameters of appropriate response to persons who suffer. Moreover, it reflects the increasingly pervasive societal unwillingness to accept that suffering is a natural and necessary part of human life.

Reviewing the Debate

In general, the debate about legalizing "aid in dying" has been limited to considerations of the scope of individual rights and self-determination; the adequacy of pain management in terminal illness; concerns about laws regulating assisted suicide and euthanasia; and the effects of proposed laws on the medical profession. Persons opposed to legalized aid in dying claim, first, that there is something unique about human life that places restrictions on individual liberty and precludes any intent and/or action to cause death. Although it is acceptable to allow death to come under certain circumstances, regard for the sanctity and dignity of human life draws the line there. Proponents counter that self-determination is the most basic of human freedoms. As death approaches, rather than place limits on a person's freedom the law should allow the broadest exercise of personal liberty. Moreover, when terminally ill persons find life unsatisfying or intolerable, failure to respond to their request for help in carrying out their freely chosen, self-destructive intentions is an affront to their dignity.

Second, seeking to dispel the fear that many persons have of pain at life's end, opponents of assisted suicide cite scientific studies that show that modern medicine has the means of relieving 90 percent of all pain, even in cases of the most advanced cancer. Moreover, they argue that fear of terminal pain can be overcome by ensuring adequate education in pain management for physicians and nurses and working to increase the awareness, availability, and use of hospice programs. Supporters of legalized aid in dying respond that the highly subjective nature of pain invalidates all such claims.

Third, opponents express concern about the ability to protect non-autonomous, gravely debilitated persons from the abuses of broadened application of this kind of legislation. Advocates reply that these concerns can be mitigated by carefully crafting the statutes to ensure inclusion of adequate safeguards.

Finally, opponents hold that the effects of this kind of legislation on individual physicians and the medical profession as a whole would be quite damaging. The only way to guard against the erosion of trust in medicine that certainly would occur if physicians were given the authority to assist persons in suicide is to maintain an absolute ban on such legislation. Defenders retort that sanctioning physician-assisted dying threatens the integrity neither of individual physicians nor of the profession. Instead, it allows physicians to provide the final step in good medical care to persons at the end of life.

Considering Suffering

Neither side in this ongoing debate about legalizing assisted suicide and euthanasia focuses appropriate attention on suffering and what should be required of members of the community in the face of suffering. Fearing that they would be relegated to the sidelines of the debate for any suggestion that some suffering simply must be accepted, opponents often avoid the topic altogether. Proponents, on the other hand, assume that persons who experience unrelieved suffering as a result of terminal illness are exempt from interpersonal responsibility and thus may break the bonds of fidelity with other members of the community. This assumption is apparent in the provision of the Oregon law that allows a terminally ill adult to choose assisted suicide without seeking counsel from family members or informing family of the decision. Some people will argue, of course, that it is precisely a sense of responsibility to family that leads the terminally ill person to seek assistance with suicide, to relieve the family of the "burden" of care.

The consistent resistance to coming to grips with the need for faithfulness among members of the human community, particularly in the face of suffering, denies basic realities about what it means to be human. First, because the human being is social by nature, every person needs and depends on the community for existence and identity. Thus, every person has a right to expect to receive what is needed for life from the community, and each person has a correlative obligation to ensure that the community is capable of supporting and nurturing life for all members. This reciprocal support is particularly important for the most basic community: the family. Second, the capacity of the community to care appropriately for persons who suffer at any stage in life depends on at least two factors. On the one hand, persons must be willing to be open to the suffering of others. Such willingness is developed over time through the experience of responding with compassion to the needs of fellow human beings. On the other hand, persons who suffer must be willing to accept the concern and care offered by others. Only through this reciprocal give and take can the community as a whole grow in its capacity to support members across the whole continuum of life.

A community that is relieved of its responsibility to care for members who experience suffering—for example, through legalized assisted suicide—risks becoming increasingly apathetic toward the needs of all members. As Dorothee Soelle points out in her work *Suffering,* this growing indifference has the capacity to destroy the community as well as the ability to form community. Soelle notes that apathy is a "social condition in which people are so dominated by the goal of avoiding suffering that it becomes a goal to avoid human relationships and contacts altogether."[2]

Finally, because the ability to create and sustain a community depends on the willingness and ability of community members to bear the burdens of one another, all members of the community have an obligation, at times, to accept and live with suffering. This final reality is certainly not widely accepted in our society. A political shift toward a "leaner and meaner" America may reflect this perspective.

Conclusion

Suffering in all its forms is an evil, and every reasonable effort should be made to relieve it. When it cannot be alleviated entirely, however, the limits of reasonableness must be set by the ongoing need to create and sustain the community of concern. Fidelity to the community will require, at times, that individual persons accept and live with suffering so that the community, now and in the future, will continue to grow in its ability to risk caring.

Notes

1. Paul Ramsey, *The Patient As Person* (New Haven, Conn.: Yale University Press, 1970), xii.

2. Dorothee Soelle, *Suffering* (Philadelphia, Penn.: Fortress Press, 1984), 36.

Chapter 58

Federal Courts Approve Physician-Assisted Suicide

Justice Clarence Thomas of the U.S. Supreme Court avowed in 1996 that when federal courts make decisions they follow precedents, "not being interested in morality."[1] When two federal appellate courts declared that physician-assisted suicide (PAS) is legal, however,[2] in an effort to strengthen their innovative opinions the courts delved into the field of morality ethics—as do most courts when they render important decisions. This chapter considers the efforts of the two courts to employ ethical concepts. Critiques of their legal argumentation are left to others.

The Second Circuit Court of Appeals tried to strengthen its argument by declaring that there is no ethical or moral difference between physician-assisted suicide and allowing a person to die when therapy is ineffective or imposes a severe burden. The reason advanced for this startling assertion is that in both cases the person in question will die, and some physical activity is needed on the part of caregivers in the dying process. Thus, the court declares that the ending of life by these means (withdrawing ineffective or burdensome life support) is nothing more or less than assisted suicide. The Ninth Circuit Court of Appeals considered the principle of double effect as a basis for its decision, maintaining that this principle enables one "to cause evil in the pursuit of good." Moreover, both decisions repeat the ethical errors of the Missouri Supreme Court insofar as the removal of artificial hydration and nutrition (AHN) is concerned, maintaining that "when Nancy Beth Cruzan's feeding and hydration tube was removed, she did not die of an underlying disease. Rather, she was allowed to starve to death." To dispel the ethical mistakes put forward by these federal appellate courts in their PAS decisions, let us consider how ethical decisions differ from physical events, the meaning of the principle of double effect, and the application of these concepts to the case of withdrawing or withholding life support, especially withdrawing AHN from a patient in a persistent vegetative state (PVS).

Principles

The essence of an ethical decision is the proximate intention (moral object) of the agent. Ethical specification into good and bad human actions does not result from observation of mere physical activity. Killing an unjust aggressor and killing an innocent person are the same insofar as physical activity is concerned, but ethically they are as different as night and day because they have different proximate intentions. In considering intention, we must realize that there are two intentions involved in every human action: the proximate intention and the remote intention. These intentions may also be called the intention of the act (proximate) and the intention of the agent (remote). The remote intention answers the question, "Why am I doing this?" The proximate intention answers the question, "What am I here and now doing in the ethical order, exclusive of my remote intention?"

Very often these intentions coincide, and the two intentions combine to form one ethical act. Sometimes, however, the intentions are different. This disjunction results in two distinct ethical specifications—one resulting from the remote intention and another resulting from the proximate intention. For example, my proximate intention may be to lead a blind man across a busy intersection. My remote intention may be to help this person. Thus, I perform an integrally good action. On the other hand, my remote intention may be to gain the confidence of the blind man so I can later defraud him of his savings. We express the relationship of the two intentions by saying, "One should not do good to achieve evil" or "The end does not justify the means."

Sometimes pursuing a proximate intention results in two distinct but necessarily connected effects. One effect is desired or intended, and the other is merely tolerated because the desired effect could not be achieved unless the unwanted effect is allowed to occur. Intending an ethically good result and merely tolerating an unwanted physical result describes the principle of double effect. A dramatic example of double effect occurs when a pregnant woman is found to have a cancerous uterus. Saving the woman's life by removing the cancerous uterus results in the death of the unborn infant. The death of the infant, because it is tolerated as a necessary physical evil is not judged in the ethical order. An effective way to judge whether one is using the principle of double effect correctly is to ask two questions: Does the good intended outweigh the evil being tolerated? and Can I truly say I would not tolerate the evil effect if it were not connected with the good effect? If the answer to both of these questions is yes, one is probably using the principle correctly.

Discussion

How do the foregoing distinctions apply to the assertions of the federal courts? The major errors of the courts are as follows:

1. They allow a good remote intention to justify an evil proximate intention. Killing an innocent person is never an ethically acceptable remote or proximate intention. Human life is a basic good, and we should never directly act in opposition to basic goods. Even though a remote intention to avoid ineffective therapy or eliminate suffering is acceptable, this remote intention should not be accomplished by a proximate intention of directly hastening death or assisting suicide. When life support is removed, the proximate intention may have two effects—one desired, the other merely tolerated. Thus, when life support is removed because it is ineffective or imposes an excessive burden, it may hasten death. The hastening of death, however, even though foreseen, is not directly intended. If a person is in a debilitated or comatose condition, the good that is achieved by removing life support far outweighs the evil that is not intended but merely tolerated.

2. In determining ethical specifications, courts consider only the physical acts, not the ethical intentions. Thus, the Second District Court of Appeals declares that omission and commission specify the ethical nature of the removal of life support, and it equates the removal of life support with killing the patient. Because the remote intention is good—relieving suffering—the end justifies evil proximate intentions such as assisting suicide.

3. Both appellate courts imply that the use of morphine or other pain-relieving analgesics intend the death of the patient. In discussing pain relief, the courts commit two errors: They mistakenly assume that the use of morphine sufficient to relieve pain will necessarily

bring about death by repressing respiration—which seldom happens. In the few cases in which pain medication does hasten death, the courts maintain that because this effect is anticipated, it is therefore intended and "causes death."

4. The viewpoint of the courts with regard to the removal of AHN is simplistic. Clearly a patient in a PVS will die if AHN is removed. Death need not be the remote or proximate intention of persons removing AHN, however. In the case of people in PVS, AHN is an ineffective therapy for the pathology that causes the permanently comatose condition, and it is burdensome as well. The proximate and remote intention would not be to kill the patient. A closer reading of the U.S. Supreme Court decision in the Cruzan case confirms that the Court did not equate removal of AHN with starving Nancy to death nor with a remote or proximate intention to cause her death, as did the Missouri Supreme Court.

Conclusion

There is no doubt that when life support is removed, we use language that could be interpreted as intending the death of the person either by remote or proximate intention. Thus, we say, "Mom will be better off dead" or "death was a blessing for dad." The meaning of these phrases, however, is not that we intend the death of mom or dad but that given the physiological condition of mom or dad, we cannot do anything beneficial for them. Thus, the proximate intention of removing life support is to discontinue ineffective therapy or to avoid excessive burden. This situation differs completely from PAS, wherein the proximate intention is to bring about the death of the patient even though the remote intention may be to eliminate suffering. Thus, removing life support from dying loved ones when it is ineffective or imposes an excessive burden is in accord with ethical norms. If death is hastened as a result of removing life support, it is merely tolerated and is the unintended price of obtaining a greater good.

Notes

1. Fred Lindecke, "Justice Plays Down Morality in Decisions," *St. Louis Post Dispatch,* May 1, 1996, 12A.
2. *Quill v. Vacco,* 2nd Federal Circuit Court of Appeals 807; 3d 713 (CA2 (N.Y.) 1996). *Compassion in Dying v. State of Washington,* 9th Federal Circuit Court of Appeals 79 Fed 3rd, 716.

Chapter 59

The U.S. Supreme Court and Assisted Suicide

"Jane Roe," a sixty-nine-year-old retired pediatrician, was diagnosed with cancer in 1988. She tried and benefitted temporarily from chemotherapy and radiation, but the cancer metastasized, and her physician referred her to hospice care. She was completely bedridden and suffered from swollen legs, poor appetite, nausea, impaired vision, bowel incontinence, and general weakness. She was mentally competent and wished to hasten her death by taking drugs prescribed by her physician. She wanted counseling and emotional support for herself and her family, as well as medical assistance at the time she would be taking the medications to end her life.

Jane Roe was one of the petitioners in a case heard by the Ninth Circuit Court of Appeals in March 1996. She died before the court issued its ruling: that the state of Washington could not prohibit physicians from prescribing life-ending medications for their mentally competent, terminally ill patients. Shortly thereafter, the Second Circuit Court of Appeals issued a similar ruling regarding a New York statute banning physician-assisted suicide. These two decisions set the stage for a June 26, 1997, ruling by the United States Supreme Court that allowed states to continue to ban physician-assisted suicide but kept the door open for future constitutional claims by dying patients.[1] This chapter examines the arguments and distinctions in the Supreme Court decision and the implications for health care professionals who care for persons with life-threatening illness.

How the Supreme Court Ruled in the Washington Case

The lower court had determined that mentally competent, terminally ill adults had a liberty right to a doctor's assistance in determining the time and manner of their death. Chief Justice William Rehnquist, in the majority opinion of the Supreme Court, interpreted the issue in the following way: Do the protections of the Fourteenth Amendment (due process) include a right to commit suicide with another's assistance? His answer was no. Rehnquist cited the following reasons for upholding a ban on assisted suicide: a 700-year history of disapproval of suicide and assisted suicide in the Anglo-American legal tradition; the state's commitment to the protection and preservation of life; state interests in protecting vulnerable people, including disabled and terminally ill people; and the danger of creating a path to voluntary and perhaps even involuntary euthanasia.

In separate concurring opinions, some justices objected to Rehnquist's formulation of the question. Justice John Paul Stevens wrote that there may be situations in which an interest in hastening death is "legitimate" and "entitled to constitutional protection." Justice Sandra Day O'Connor said that although there is no "generalized right" to commit suicide, the narrower question is whether a mentally competent person who is experiencing great suffering has a constitutional interest in controlling the circumstances of his or her imminent death. According to O'Connor, there is no need to address this issue because patients in Washington can obtain palliative care, even when doing so would indirectly hasten their deaths. She concludes that the ban on assisted suicide is justified by the difficulty in defining terminal illness and the risk that a dying patient's request for assistance might not be truly voluntary.

How the Supreme Court Ruled
in the New York Case

The lower court had ruled that terminally ill persons who aren't attached to life support should be allowed to hasten their deaths by self-administering prescribed drugs because New York law also permits a terminally ill, mentally competent person to refuse life-sustaining treatment. In the view of the lower court, ending life by withdrawing life support is no different than assisted suicide. Rehnquist wrote that "unlike the Court of Appeals, we think the distinction between assisting suicide and withdrawing life-sustaining treatment, a distinction widely recognized and endorsed in the medical profession and in our legal traditions, is both important and logical; it is certainly rational." Ethics and the law have long recognized the distinction between causation and intent. When a patient refuses life-sustaining medical treatment, she or he dies from the underlying fatal pathology or disease. If a patient ingests lethal medication prescribed by a physician, he or she is killed by the medication. A doctor who provides painkilling drugs may hasten a patient's death, but the physician's purpose and intent may be to ease the patient's pain. A doctor who assists a suicide must intend primarily that the patient be made dead. The Supreme Court rightly recognized that intention is ethically relevant in distinguishing between two acts that may have the same result.

Implications for Health Care Professionals

The Supreme Court strongly suggested that state legislatures are the proper venues for action regarding assisted suicide. In a lengthy concurring opinion, Justice David Souter argued that states have superior opportunities to obtain the facts necessary for a judgment about doctor-assisted suicide. He noted that states can experiment, move forward, and pull back as facts emerge within their jurisdictions. Only one state, Oregon, has voted to permit physician-assisted suicide. Situating the public debate in the states provides an opportunity for health care professionals, individually and collectively, to address the real issue: inadequate care for people at the end of life.

The assisted suicide controversy challenges health care professionals to transform the way we care for persons who are dying. Our efforts to relieve suffering and alleviate symptoms are insufficient. Pain management is rarely taught in medical schools, and palliative care is not a recognized specialty in the United States. A common misconception of palliative care is that it focuses solely on keeping people "comfortable." Appropriate care for persons who are dying blends the science of pain management with a focus on emotional and spiritual care that reaches far beyond the traditional realm of medicine.

One critical issue is how we might finance palliative care. Medicare has no reimbursement category for patients who are dying, although the federal government is testing such as category. Health care professionals have an ethical obligation to advocate for more integrated and better financed care for the dying.

Conclusion

In 1997 a coalition of six Catholic health care organizations formed Supportive Care of the Dying: A Coalition of Compassionate Care.[2] These organizations conducted a systematic study of the needs and experiences of individuals with life-threatening illness, their families, their caregivers, and their communities. The study's findings argue for reform of the care provided to persons who are facing death. Life-threatening illness is more than a medical event, and care at the end of life requires a partnership between the health care system and the community. The coalition recommends that health care organizations fund programs that promote community-based healing; create managed-care organizations that recognize that people cope with life-threatening illness as members of a community; improve hospice programs through provider training; and replace provider-centered protocols with patient-centered care.

Nothing would have changed the ultimate result of Jane Roe's cancer. However, we might have alleviated her pain, relieved her symptoms, and addressed her suffering in more skilled and compassionate ways. The real issue is not whether there is a constitutional or legislative "right to die" but how well we care for persons with life-threatening illness, their families, their caregivers, and their communities.

Notes

1. U.S. Supreme Court, *Vacco v. Quill*, reversed, 521 U.S. 793 117 S.Ct.2293, 138 L.Ed. 2nd 834. (6/26/97).
2. U.S. Supreme Court, *Washington v. Glucksberg*, reversed, 521, U.S. 793, 117 S.Ct.2293, 138, L.Ed. 2nd 834.

Chapter 60

Social Aspects of Assisted Suicide

On August 15, 1996, forty-two-year-old Judith Curren, who suffered from chronic fatigue syndrome, killed herself with the help of Jack Kevorkian. According to Kevorkian's attorney, Mrs. Curren had been required to undergo family counseling and psychiatric evaluation prior to her suicide.[1] Nevertheless, at the time of the procedure Kevorkian was unaware that Mrs. Curren had filed assault charges against her husband about a month previously.

Three general questions arising in this case deserve our attention: Why is an understanding of the social milieu an important factor in decisions about assisted suicide? Is it ethically permissible (or even possible) to make a "substantively independent" decision to commit assisted suicide? What are the social implications of decisions to commit assisted suicide?

Principles

It is a well-established tenet of good medicine that health care providers must obtain an adequate social history before they can competently assist a patient with important medical decisions. This maxim rests on two considerations. First, a good social history can alert a clinician to factors that threaten a patient's autonomy, such as undue social pressure from family members, associates, or friends. Second, the social history is a means by which clinicians come to understand their patients as distinct persons, embedded in a web of family and cultural relationships. Every patient has a story, and every story is rife with social detail—full of loyalties, rivalries, antagonisms, sympathies, and ambitions. Only amidst these relations can we situate our patients. Only here can we identify the nexus of social obligations and responsibilities that have an important influence in equitable decision making.

In an age of patient rights and sometimes exaggerated claims about the implications of the ethical principle of autonomy, we often neglect the fact that patients have responsibilities. We behave as if patients exist in a state of social isolation, unencumbered by the normal constraints of community. From this perspective, the aim of medicine is simply to serve the stated preferences of each patient. Yet occasionally—as when a patient requests parenteral narcotics and also insists on driving—we are forced to retreat from this untenable position.

In the case of Judith Curren, the social history—or the way it was applied—was inadequate because it failed to serve either of the aforementioned functions. The fact that Mrs. Curren had recently charged her psychiatrist husband with assault indicates the likelihood of significant marital disharmony. Kevorkian's ignorance about this episode suggests that he may not have taken adequate steps to ensure that her decision was uncoerced. The second consideration, however, seems more important in this matter, both for the evaluation of the Curren case and for the issue of assisted suicide in general. Did Dr. Kevorkian take adequate stock of Judith Curren's social needs and responsibilities?

Discussion

The principle of autonomy holds a central place in medical ethics. This principle requires that patients be allowed (and, if necessary, helped) to make decisions independently. The meaning of "independently" is a matter for debate. Gerald Dworkin distinguishes "procedural independence," which is achieved in practices such as obtaining routine informed consent, from "substantive independence." The latter is independence in its purest state and is, for Dworkin, a lofty ideal. Dworkin holds that substantive independence is incompatible with loyalty, love, or compassion because these attributes "are to some extent determined by the needs and predicaments of others."[2]

Conceiving the principle of autonomy in terms of "substantive independence" is undesirable for two reasons: Autonomous actions, under such a principle, would be impossible, and a conception of autonomy that excludes factors such as loyalty and love severs ethics from its foundation in human experience. Substantive independence requires that our decisions and actions are entirely our own. Clearly this ideal is impossible because we speak and think using socially acquired linguistic signs, laden with the values of our intellectual ancestors. Our personal aims are even more prone to the influence of others because they generally derive largely from our membership in one social group or another. Even automatic, unthinking actions are socially conditioned to a degree, as Pavlov and Skinner have demonstrated. Substantive independence is incompatible with the experience of being human.

This incompatibility is not merely an existential liability; it is also an ethical one. Most contemporary ethicists believe that ethics aims at human flourishing and that human knowledge must be sought in human experience. This position does not imply we are all secular humanists: Most theologians hold that God is manifest in human experience, including divine revelation. It does imply, however, that any justifiable ethical principle of autonomy will reflect the manner in which thriving human beings actually behave. One of the universally recognized aspects of such human ethical experience is that it manifests the aforementioned attributes of loyalty, love, and compassion.

As Aristotle observed, the human being is a social animal. To thrive we need more than food and shelter, work and rest. We need affiliations. We need to live in communities, and to live fruitfully within communities we must honor the values and ideals that animate and define these communities. As thinkers such as Josiah Royce have painstakingly demonstrated, this imperative undergirds the health of each individual. It is a psychological need as well as an ethical one. Thus, in satisfying our social needs, we take on social responsibilities. These responsibilities are not merely the price we pay for the benefits of dwelling within a community; they are themselves the primary benefits of membership. Our social commitments allow us to formulate coherent and satisfying life plans and, ultimately, to forge our personal identities.

A workable ethical principle of autonomy recognizes that the independence of each individual depends on these social prerequisites. Any action—including assisted suicide—is independent in a morally acceptable sense only when it coheres with the fundamental, socially conditioned moral commitments of the moral agent.

Conclusion

Several actual or potential implications of Judith Curren's assisted suicide weigh against the procedure. First, it contributes to the inauguration of social norms that could powerfully influence future estimates of self-worth and the desirability of living. Consider the social pressures affecting chronically ill persons who believe they are a burden to their families: What if such a person lived in a family in which healthier members praised and esteemed a relative who had opted for assisted suicide? Suppose such a person lived in a neighborhood where someone like Mrs. Curren was idolized for a "courageous" decision to commit suicide. To believe that decisions about assisted suicide exist in a vacuum, affecting only the patient, is to subscribe to a naive social psychology.

A second implication is difficult to analyze in Judith Curren's case because it would require details about her social life that are unavailable. Mrs. Curren was probably a contributing member of various small and large communities. What were the effects of her suicide for these communities that supported Judith Curren and, in turn, relied on her support?

Third, Mrs. Curren's suicide establishes a precedent that non-life-threatening illnesses associated with minimal to moderate physical debilitation may be acceptable medical indications for suicide. Such an approach is inconsistent with the integrity of medicine, based on its own self-understanding. Certainly medicine is committed to the alleviation of suffering. Yet it is also committed to preserving human life when this life holds the promise of future human fulfillment and to avoiding harm.[3] Chronic fatigue syndrome does not preclude human fulfillment. Furthermore, there are manifold ways in which Mrs. Curren's suffering could have been mitigated without harming her physically.

Finally, I lack confidence that Jack Kevorkian—or anyone—is insightful enough to guarantee that Judith Curren was not betraying her own deepest moral commitments by fleeing her medical problems. She likely suffered physical and emotional pain that was deep enough to cloud her perception of social opportunities and hinder her capacity to evaluate and judge her social needs. A compassionate health care provider would attend, first and foremost, to these incapacities.

Notes

1. "Kevorkian Brings 2 Bodies to Hospital within Eight Hours," *St. Louis Post-Dispatch,* August 23, 1996.
2. Gerald Dworkin, "Autonomy and Behavior Control," *Hastings Center Report* 6 (February 1976): 26.
3. Albert R. Jonsen, Mark Siegler, and William J. Winslade, *Clinical Ethics,* 4th ed. (New York: McGraw-Hill, 1998), 141.

Chapter 61 _____

Can Liberty Sustain Itself? Reflections on Physician-Assisted Suicide

"Give me liberty or give me death." Patrick Henry's words have stimulated the American imagination for our nation's entire history. Although we often think of laws as restricting liberties, the American passion for liberty has been a driving force in the development of our laws and recognized rights. Perhaps the greatest area of development in our legal tradition during the twentieth century has been in the realm of protecting the right to religious freedom and the "unenumerated" right to privacy. Although a right to privacy was fairly well entrenched in the civil law of most states by the mid-1930s, it was explicitly recognized for the first time in a Supreme Court decision in *Griswold v.*

Connecticut.[1] Invoking the right to privacy, the Court prohibited a ban on the use of birth control substances within marriage. The rationale behind this ruling was not that people had a state-given or human right to practice birth control per se; the idea was that a law is bad if its enforcement requires the state to enter the bedrooms of married couples. The right to privacy has always been closely connected with the right to liberty. In this case, the connection involved primarily a freedom from invasion into a private domain.

Since 1965, however, the concept of a right to privacy has slowly developed into something of a freedom to—that is, it has come to be regarded as a more positive right, so that anything we do that we consider private or intimate (e.g., anything in the realm of sexuality or religion) is beyond the reach of the law. Of course, this sort of logic cannot be—and normally is not—carried out to its logical extreme. If it were, it would protect all sorts of sexual abuse or religious acts involving human sacrifice. Naturally, other significant competing goods may provide constraints on the rights to privacy and liberty—But what sorts of goods?

In *Washington v. Glucksberg,*[2] the Supreme Court considered the claim that an absolute prohibition of physician-assisted suicide violated the Fourteenth Amendment insofar as it unduly restricted the liberties of some Americans, particularly in the private and intimate realm of death. The plaintiffs felt that they were in a particularly strong position to argue the case because in *Planned Parenthood v. Casey* (1993) the Court had insisted that at "the heart of liberty is the right to define one's own concept of existence, of meaning, of the universe, and of the mystery of human life." To the disappointment of many defenders of liberty, the Supreme Court in *Glucksberg* ruled that there was no fundamental liberty interest at stake and that the state's interests in prohibiting physician-assisted suicide are rational. The Court also made clear, however, that there is nothing in the U.S. Constitution prohibiting assisted suicide. Thus, the debate may continue at a state level, and well-framed laws permitting assisted suicide may be upheld by the Supreme Court. To date, physician-assisted suicide is legal in only one state, Oregon, though legislation is pending in other states. The recent case of *Krischer v. McIver* in Florida made amply clear that the argument for assisted suicide based on an appeal to a right to privacy is still operative. How could it not be, when this concept cuts to the heart of our American identity?

Constraining Liberty to Preserve Liberty

What sorts of goods may provide constraints on our liberty rights, even in the private realm? At a minimum, *goods that are needed to guarantee lib-*

erty may also constrain liberty. In trying to identify the goods that are needed to preserve liberty, a brief psychological digression is in order. This digression is necessary because liberty is first and foremost a feature of human beings with a certain psychological makeup; thus, any jurisprudence of liberty that wishes to be adequate will need to take this makeup into account.

Viktor Frankl, the founder of "logotherapy," posited the existence of a central principle that guides human action, as his Viennese predecessors, Sigmund Freud and Alfred Adler had done. Freud initially suggested that the guiding principle was the "pleasure principle;" Adler suggested that it was the "will to power." Frankl suggested that the guiding principle is the "will to meaning"—a fundamental urge to find meaning in one's concrete life situation, to find a *reason* to be happy and to live. Frankl's most famous book, *Man's Search for Meaning,* describes his central psychological thesis in the context of his experiences in several Nazi concentration camps (where he lost his first wife, parents, and siblings).[3] It is not surprising that a psychiatrist who lived through the Nazi regime did not restrict his reflection on psychological pathologies to the individual but also looked at these pathologies as they affect society.

Decades after Frankl's Holocaust experience, he tells the story of an encounter with a taxi driver in the United States who asserted that the present generation is mad: "They kill themselves, they kill each other, and they take dope." This statement exemplifies what Frankl came to call the triad of collective neuroses: depression, aggression, and addiction. Individually or collectively, we develop neuroses—in part, Frankl says, when we lose sight of transcendent goods that lend meaning to our lives and when we lose the belief that *all life under all conditions* (e.g., nearly starved and ill in a Nazi concentration camp) has meaning. Everyone knows that neuroses—more specifically, afflictions such as depression, antisocial disorders, or substance dependence—deprive persons of liberty: They make it harder to act at all, harder to act civilly, and harder to act according to one's own will, respectively.

The "Philosopher's Brief"—*an amicus curiae* brief submitted to the Supreme Court in *Washington v. Glucksberg*—provided perhaps the most powerful justification of physician-assisted suicide in terms of a liberty right (arguing that one's death is intimate, personal, and in the realm of private morality).[4] The authors of that brief suggest that suicide should not be an option in cases in which it would not be rational. One example of an irrational suicide would be the otherwise healthy person who acts out of a severe depression over his or her unrequited love. In such a case, they say, we might well expect the person later to be grateful that his or her liberty to commit suicide was restricted. They do not observe, however, that in permitting some cases of suicide, one must assume that it is *not reasonable* to expect some persons to be grateful for their life—that is, one assumes that there are some cases in which it is *reasonable* to maintain that life is no longer meaningful. It is important to take note of this fact because people often assume that by being permissive the state remains neutral, whereas in prohibiting it takes a moral stance. This analysis, however, is simply naive. In permitting and in prohibiting, the state takes a stance and reinforces certain ideas. The debate is always over which ideas to reinforce and what impact this stance will have on the common good.

Conclusion

We love liberty, but our liberty is in fact restricted when we become depressed, antisocial, or addicted. Frankl suggests that we are predisposed to these psychological disorders when we lose faith that life is meaningful under all circumstances. It would seem to follow that if we love liberty, we must protect certain fundamental beliefs and goods that ensure its existence. Although this kind of argument may be quite different from those typically considered by federal and state judges, it ought to be given serious attention by everyone who loves liberty—especially by those who are asked to act upon a naive logic of liberty. Physicians and all health care workers have a professional obligation to come to the aid of people who are dying and in great pain. In the end, however, high-quality palliative care and psychological support will best serve the individual patient; insofar as they also reinforce a healthy conviction about human life, they also will best serve the common good.

Notes

1. See Michael J. Sandel, "Moral Argument and Liberal Toleration," *California Law Review* 77 (1989): 521–38.
2. 505 U.S. at 851, 1996.
3. See Viktor Frankl, *Man's Search for Meaning: An Introduction to Logotherapy* (Boston: Beacon Press, 1992).
4. "Assisted Suicide: The Philosophers' Brief," *New York Review of Books,* May 21, 1997, 41–47.

Part Eight

Managed Care

Chapter 62

Ethical Issues and Managed Care: Asking the Right Questions

Beginning a discussion of ethical issues raised by managed care with a brief consideration of language is instructive. In the past, words used to modify "care" gave some indication of the health-related needs of persons. Thus, "critical," "acute," "long-term," "hospice," and other words have been used to describe a level or approach to care based on health needs. When the word "managed" is used to modify care, however, quite another reality is conveyed. The term *managed care* indicates a focus not on the needs of persons whose health is at risk but on the needs of payers and providers (individual, corporate, governmental, and others) who are concerned about cost. This claim is verified by reviewing the many definitions of managed care in the literature. For example: "Managed care is a system that, in varying degrees, integrates the financing and delivery of medical care through contracts with selected physicians and hospitals. All forms of managed care represent attempts to control costs by modifying the behavior of doctors."[1] In itself, the shift in focus from persons seeking care to persons and organizations providing care may not be highly significant. However, it should alert anyone who is concerned about the ethical integrity of our health care system to the need for constant vigilance and, in particular, of the need to raise the correct questions.

The seemingly endless stream of articles being written today about the ethical issues raised by managed care focus almost exclusively on the potential effects it may have on the patient-physician relationship. Authors ask questions such as, What effect will financial incentives have

239

on a physician's decisions about treatment options for a given patient? How will trust be maintained in the relationship when the patient realizes that the physician/employee of a large health maintenance organization (HMO) may have divided loyalties? How can the gatekeeper physician ensure that patients are adequately informed about alternatives not covered under a health plan so that they can purchase them outside the plan? Although these concerns are important, focusing exclusively on such issues is myopic and misleading. This narrow view gives the impression that ethical concerns are raised by the structure or functional components of managed care itself. This impression, in turn, leads to the conclusion that shoring up the structure with practice rules and guidelines, outcome studies, and quality indicators will ensure the ethical integrity of managed care as a delivery mechanism.

Two points should be noted in considering ethical questions about managed care. First, managed care itself is neither morally good nor bad. It is simply a vehicle, a means to an end, and thus in itself is morally neutral. Second, the risks that managed care poses to the good of persons (i.e., ethical concerns) arise primarily because of the context within which managed care is being adopted. That context includes the attitudes, practices, and beliefs of persons who use managed care as a means to a desired goal. Thus, asking relevant questions about the ethical issues raised by managed care must begin with an appropriate understanding of the context within which it is spreading.

Context

Managed care has been part of the U.S. health care system for several decades. It has only recently gained prominence as a preferred way to deliver and finance health care services. During the recent debate about health care reform, managed care has been promoted as an effective and efficient way to deliver quality health services while containing costs. Proponents have argued that widespread adoption of managed care would help to accomplish the goals of systemic reform when accompanied by guaranteed universal access, employer mandates, and premium caps. The problem, of course, is that when the reform effort failed the accompanying pieces—which were intended to ensure the integrity of managed care within the new system—were abandoned. The possibility of retrieving any of them seems remote in the present environment.

There are at least four fundamental reasons for the failure of reform and the rejection of universal access, employer mandates, and premium caps.

First, there was no social consensus on the question of a right to basic health care for all persons. The radical individualism so characteristic of our contemporary society found expression in the frequently aired "Harry and Louise" commercials sponsored by opponents of reform. This white, middle-class couple convinced many Americans of all ages and ilks that reform would have only negative effects on their exercise of individual freedom. The proposal to radically reform the system and level the playing field to ensure fair access to needed services for all persons gave way to speculation about long waiting lines, limited access to expensive and exotic interventions, and higher health care premiums to cover the cost of care for the poor. Concern about promoting the common good—a foundational principle central to the reform effort—fell to the battle cry of "my rights" and "me first!" Second, there was no political will to challenge people who argued on behalf of individual rights and liberties over the needs of the community or the nation. Various interest groups made it quite clear that legislators who did so would find themselves seeking other employment after the next election. Third, neither Congress nor any public group had the strength to effectively constrain the powerful interests of the insurance industry and other self-interested players. Thus, any suggestion that a truly reformed and therefore just system must include budgets, premium caps, and reasonable limits on profits went down with the ship. Attempts to salvage them appears to be a futile effort. Fourth, there was little or no recognition among legislators or the public that substantive reform required a significant challenge to the values that inform and drive social institutions such as health care.

Thus, values such as individualism and consumerism that have undermined meaningful reform efforts in the past remain within the system and undoubtedly will continue to have negative effects on the system in the future. It is surprising that managed care is spreading in this context because it is a mechanism intended to place some restrictions on the very things that many of the opponents of health care reform hold dear. It is troubling that managed care is being adopted widely in this environment because it is susceptible to the same distortions, excesses, and injustices that have been so harmful and difficult to deal with in the past. As values such as individualism and consumerism and the attitudes and behaviors they breed inevitably find expression in managed care, they do so under the influence of other powerful factors. These other factors include the increasingly negative and often punitive rhetoric that accompanies discussions about reforming the welfare system or managing issues of intergenerational justice, and the growing sense of xenophobia that appears to be sweeping the country and is embodied in legislation such as Proposition 187 in California.

Raising the Ethical Questions

In this environment, asking the right questions about managed care is essential. For example, it is not sufficient to ask questions about how to ensure that the incentives offered to physicians to limit unnecessary interventions do not lead to undertreatment. A more fundamental question should be raised: Must we simply acquiesce to the proposal that incentives of any sort must be part of the structure of the evolving health care system? In particular, must we accept as appropriate incentives that are designed to contain costs by influencing physician practice patterns? The mere acceptance of such incentives as reasonable strikes at the heart of the medical and other health professions. Acceptance legitimates the further demise of altruism as a requisite character trait for physicians and others. It fosters the popular perception that self-interest is appropriate as a primary motive for members of the healing professions. Our questions should reflect a recognition that it was precisely the acceptance of self-interest as consistent with professionalism that gave rise to much of the abuse in the fee-for-service approach to health care that we are now seeking so ardently to reform.

It is not sufficient to ask how to market and advertise a managed care product so that it does not discourage certain persons or categories of persons from seeking admission. A more fundamental question must be asked: How can we ensure that the dignity of every person is adequately respected regardless of the impact that his or her health status or socioeconomic situation may have on the bottom line? How can we guarantee that a Medicaid or Medicare HMO does not reflect inadvertently the growing resentment that many people in our society harbor against poor or elderly persons?

Conclusion

Two important considerations should guide us as we develop more probing and focused questions about managed care in an effort to ensure that care is delivered in an ethical manner. First, managed care is merely a vehicle, a means to an end. Second, good people give good care.

Note

1. John Inglehart, "Physicians and the Growth of Managed Care," *New England Journal of Medicine* 331, no. 17 (October 27, 1994): 1167–71.

Chapter 63

Harry and Louise: What Happened?

As the Clinton administration was planning a total reorganization of health care in the United States, "Harry and Louise" appeared in a series of television advertisements sponsored by the Health Insurance Association of America. Harry and Louise discussed the plans for the renewal of health care in the United States and lamented that "there must be a better way." The implication of these vignettes was twofold: one, that increased government involvement in health care would elevate the cost of health care, limit access to health care, dilute the quality of health care, enmesh health care in a crippling bureaucracy, and make it much more difficult to visit a physician of one's choice; and two, that all of these issues would be handled more expediently and effectively if market forces and private enterprise were allowed to control the provision of health care.

Harry and Louise misled us, however. After plans to increase the presence of the federal government in health care were defeated and abandoned, market forces and private enterprise have been allowed to dominate the provision of health care provided by private agencies. Indeed, even programs financed by the federal government, such as Medicare and Medicaid, are gradually adapting health maintenance organizations and other mechanisms developed to maximize the effect of market forces. The new methods of providing and financing health care have not brought solutions to the problems besetting heath care, however. More than forty million people in the United States still do not have adequate access to health care. Moreover, although cost escalation has been controlled, at least temporarily, the overall cost of health care has not been reduced. Health care seems to be getting more expensive for individuals because of deductible insurance policies. If health care insurance companies' dreams become reality, coverage for health care will require more direct contributions on the part of patients. In addition, permission to obtain health care has become more enmeshed in a bureaucratic morass; utilization review often requires the permission of a bureaucrat who is far distant from therapeutic decisions. Finally, the very nature of health care is challenged by market forces that treat health care as a commodity.

The methods used to modify health care practices in the name of market effectiveness are well known. Fundamentally, they involve the manipulation of physicians and hospitals by insurance companies so that they are "persuaded" to charge less for their services and to offer fewer services. Thus, Harry and Louise were in error. Can we learn anything from this error?

The problem with introducing market forces into the provision of health care is twofold:

- Market forces do not have any concern for poor and aging persons in our society. Poor and aging persons do not have power to influence the market because they are not producers.
- Market forces offer some hope of limiting and reducing costs and promoting quality if all participants are equal in the market. If one group has a monopoly, however, market forces are beneficial only for the group enjoying monopolistic powers.

If we posit that three groups participate in the health care market—patients, providers, and payors—the payors (that is, the insurance corporations) seem to have a monopoly. Although hospitals as providers are also affected by the monopolistic powers of insurance companies, this chapter focuses on the response of physicians. How can physicians offset the tendency toward monopolistic practice on the part of the insurers?

Some physicians, are forming labor unions to limit the power of insurance companies. Many more are joining with other physicians in group practices, and some are uniting with hospitals to protect their interests. Although some unified response to health insurance regulations on the part of physicians is justified, the labor union is not the proper model for that response. Labor unions, especially in recent times, have been concerned mainly with one thing: increased wages for union members. If physicians adopt a model of response that bespeaks concern mainly about their own salaries, they will destroy the public trust that is so vital for the profession of medicine.

Instead, the model for physician response to the power of insurance companies should be the guild—which flourished in the Middle Ages as civic communities developed. Artisans and craftsmen came together in guilds to improve their economic conditions, but they realized that their economic well-being depended on the quality of their products and that they could not carry on their trades and crafts unless peace was present in society. Thus, although the economic interests of guild members was of concern, this concern was subordinate to the desire to provide quality products and to protect the common good of the community. The guilds flourished for many years. Many of them formed ethical codes for their professional practice. Often, guilds would be able to elect some of their members directly to governing bodies in the community, thereby demonstrating their concern for the common good. Guilds were often accused of limiting competition. This claim was partially true, but partially untrue. Mainly, competition was limited in the name of quality production. The competency of people introduced into the trade or craft, and thus introduced into the guild, was controlled. The limitation on the number of people admitted to the guild was not totally for self-serving reasons, however.

Applying the guild concept to the present situation in health care would not be difficult. Physicians should offer unified opposition to the regulations of insurance companies if the regulations are truly detrimental to quality care of patients. Yet simply because a regulation changes the way medicine has been practiced or provided in the past does not mean that the change is detrimental to patient well-being. Changes are needed in the manner in which health care has been provided for the past twenty-five years. There must be an honest evaluation of the changes, however. The norm for evaluation is not profit for payors or providers but patient benefit.

Physicians have a narrow row to hoe to avoid the image of being self-serving. When the Clinton administration called together hundreds of "experts" to redesign the financing and provision of health care, there were no physicians in the group. Can you imagine a reform of the courts being designed without the active participation of lawyers? Although the fact that physicians were not included was outrageous, even more significant from a social point of view was the fact that there was little public opposition or indignation resulting from the exclusion. Was the lack of opposition to the exclusion of physicians from the Clinton bargaining table an indication that the general public believes that physicians seek their own economic benefit exclusively, oblivious to professional responsibility or the well-being of patients?

Conclusion

Changes are needed in the provision of health care. Many people are excluded from adequate access to health care. Moreover, some changes endanger the practice of good medicine. Physicians as a group must lead the effort to benefit patients—and in so doing, benefit themselves.

Chapter 64 _____

Managed Care and Early Discharge of Newborn Infants

A study published in the August 1996 issue of *Pediatrics* suggested that sending full-term babies home from the hospital less than 48 hours after birth poses no danger to their survival chances.[1] Researchers in Utah concluded that most full-term newborns who died showed symptoms of their difficulties within 18 hours after birth. These results added fuel to the debate over "drive-through" childbirths, in which mothers and newborns are discharged from the hospital 24 hours or less after a vaginal delivery and 48 hours or less after a cesarean delivery. Such early discharges have become *common* in the era of cost-cutting. Physicians and mothers often oppose the practice, saying that it takes at least two days for mothers to recover and to ensure that their babies are healthy.

In response to public demand, President Clinton signed the Mothers and Newborns Health Protection Act, which was sponsored by Senators Bill Bradley and Nancy Kassebaum. This legislation required insurance companies to cover at least 48 hours of inpatient care for mothers and infants after a vaginal delivery and 96 hours after a cesarean delivery. At least twenty-eight states have passed similar laws giving patients and physicians more flexibility in determining an appropriate length of stay after childbirth.

How did the most fundamental of nature's events become the center of such heated controversy? Why are women and children the focus of the first major public debate over managed care? To examine the ethical issues involved in this discussion, this chapter considers the impact of managed care on patients' trust in medical care and in their physicians, the balance of medical and economic judgments, and the use of government mandates to address single issues of care.

Principles

Trust has always been central to the relationships between physicians and patients. The success of medical care depends on patients' trust that their physicians are competent, take appropriate responsibility and control, and give their patients' welfare the highest priority. Trust enables patients to communicate private information and place their health—indeed their lives—in the hands of their physicians. Managed care arrangements that restrict choice or dictate medical decisions potentially challenge the ability of physicians to sustain trust.

The goal of caring for patients serves as the foundation of ethical medical practice. Patients generally expect their physicians to be dedicated first and foremost to serving their needs for quality care. Yet the American Medical Association's current Principles of Medical Ethics state that physicians are responsible not only to their patients but also to society, to other health care professionals, and to themselves. Economic factors are especially prominent today with the national focus on cost-containment and efficient use of finite resources. Ethical physicians must balance economic judgments and decisions about medical care.

Ideally, social decisions should be made by persons who experience and are most strongly affected by the decisions concerning them. Decisions about health care, for example, pertain most not to government but to bodies of physicians and patients who are mutually dependent on each other. The role of government is to coordinate and encourage the full development of the different organs of society, not to deprive them of their decision-making capacity. Governments and bureaucratic organizations are not likely to personalize the health care they give. Decision making should be shared by everyone concerned, in mutual interdependence.[2]

Discussion

Good ethics begins with good data. Let us examine the historical development and results of research with mothers and newborns in early-discharge programs. Kaiser Permanente initiated the first early-discharge program in 1976 in response to demand from patients. No complications were believed to be related to early discharge (defined as 12 hours after normal delivery), and patient satisfaction was very high. Interestingly, substantial cost savings were not achieved. Subsequent small studies suggested that discharge before 48 hours for a vaginal birth may be safe for selected populations at low risk, with careful antenatal screening and multiple postpartum visits. No adequately designed studies have examined early discharge with comprehensive post-discharge services. Early discharge has particular implications for breastfeeding and the treatment of jaundice and sepsis. Appropriate education to allow new mothers to develop confidence in breastfeeding is critical, but substantial milk production does not occur until the second to fourth postpartum day.

Not surprisingly, insurers want to discharge mothers and newborns as quickly as possible. They estimate that shortening the length of stay by 24 hours could save $4 billion without causing lasting harm to mothers or children. Length of stay had already fallen from four days in 1970 to two days in 1992 for all vaginal births and from eight to four days for all cesarean deliveries. Health plan administrators claim that the long hospitalizations of the past were unnecessary for mothers and children.

The primary motivation for early-discharge programs, however, is not to benefit mothers and children but to enable health care insurers to retain more premium dollars. Thus, quality, safety, and medical necessity become secondary to cost in judging the effectiveness of programs. Collaborative decision making between physicians and patients is undermined and physicians are held hostage to the dictates of third-party payers. If we are to preserve trust and advocacy as the basis of the patient-physician relationship, we must balance medical judgments about safety and quality with economic judgments about efficient use of resources.

In 1995, the American Academy of Pediatrics (AAP) set forth medical criteria for discharge after childbirth. AAP said that length of stay is best based on an assessment of the health of the mother and the baby as a pair, home support, and the surety of follow-up. The timing of discharge should be determined by physicians caring for the infant, not by an arbitrary policy established by third-party payers. AAP recognizes that it generally takes more than 48 hours to meet the criteria for discharge, and it encourages efforts to keep mothers and infants together until they are ready to go home. Guidelines such as these should determine insurance reimbursement. Government intervention may be necessary if insurers will not honor professional guidelines and physician judgment. The federal legislation does not force women to stay in the hospital. It puts decision making back into the hands of physicians by requiring health plans and insurance companies to cover care that is consistent with AAP's professional medical guidelines. Although reform is laudatory, we cannot solve the real or perceived problems of market-driven medicine by passing statutes dealing with single issues of care. It would be wiser to require all insurers to offer the same basic benefits package to all subscribers.

Conclusion

The fact that a 48-hour stay can be accomplished does not mean that it is appropriate for every mother and infant. Respect for persons demands that patients be treated as people in need of care, not customers in need of management. We must implement managed care techniques in a way that protects patients and the integrity of the patient-physician relationship. Physicians should follow established professional guidelines to determine the appropriate length of stay for women and infants after childbirth. More stringent or more lenient guidelines could be used at the discretion of the physician.

Perhaps we have a failure of the imagination here. The early Kaiser program was developed in response to demand from women who wanted to spend less time in the hospital after childbirth. We need conclusive research to demonstrate whether the necessary monitoring and education could be done as effectively and efficiently by visiting nurses who specialize in newborn care at home. Physicians, patients, and insurers could then work together to ensure that post-discharge services are available for women and infants as soon as they are ready to go home.

Notes

1. "Survival of Drive-Through Babies Same as Others—Study," *American Medical News* (September 2, 1996), 11.
2. David Mechanic and Mark Scheslinger, "The Impact of Managed Care on Patients' Trust In Medical Care and Their Physicians," *JAMA* 275 (June 5, 1996): 1693.

Chapter 65 _____

Treating Symptoms or Basic Causes

Anyone who lives on the far side of the moon may not have heard of the changes occurring in health care. The majority of the population, however, realizes that the provision and financing of health care has changed considerably. The days when health care was offered by individuals or stand-alone facilities are past. Corporations now dominate the provision of health care. Not only are physicians and acute-care facilities assimilated into corporations; corporations now offer home health care and hospice care as well. Scores of articles have been published in prominent health care journals seeking to analyze the new developments resulting from the phenomenon of increased corporate provision of health care. Although most of these articles list only the harmful effects of corporate activity, there are good effects as well. Moreover, most of the articles suggest counteracting harmful effects by means of legislation. Although some legislation may be helpful, legislation treats only the symptoms, not the fundamental causes. This chapter attempts to recognize some of the beneficial effects of corporate health care and offers more fundamental norms than legislation for counteracting the harmful effects of corporate health care.

Principles

Most of the aforementioned articles seem to use the term "managed care" to designate all of the unpopular or harmful innovations introduced by corporate health care in the past ten years. In fact, managed care, or corporate care, is not all bad. As one prominent physician states:

> The inherent virtues of managed care have manifested themselves in many salutary improvements to the system that might otherwise never have been made. These include attempts to eliminate waste and redundancy, a greater focus on health promotion and disease prevention, more attention to the management of chronic diseases, a focus on the accountability of physicians and health plans on the quality of care, lower hospitalization rates without an obvious decline in the quality of care, heavy investment in patient information systems and control of employer health care costs.[1]

A second characteristic of the articles evaluating corporate or managed care is that they overlook significant problems in our health care system. A viable and mutually beneficial health care system requires that the ultimate goal of the system must be the well-being of all citizens, not generating a profit for stockholders. Clearly, to maintain a viable presence, all health corporations must generate an excess of income over expenditures; health care professionals and administrators must receive a just salary. Yet the notion that people not connected with health care should make money, or even become wealthy, as the result of investments that depend on illness and the suffering of others is reprehensible.

The obstacle preventing a beneficent and just health care system is best illustrated by the phrase "investor-owned" health care corporations. This phrase conveys the notion that all practices of health care corporations are to be governed by market forces. Of course, the market has no concern for vulnerable people, no matter what the source of their vulnerability. Many representatives of investor-owned health care corporations would respond to the foregoing statement by saying, "We seek to do both; we provide quality health care and make a profit at the same time." The problem with this argument is that in human affairs we always direct our endeavors to one ultimate goal. Jesus stated this truth in the words, "No one can serve two masters." It is possible to have an intermediate goal of making a profit with an ultimate goal of providing services to people and still provide beneficent health care. If profit is the ultimate goal, however, sooner or later service will be sacrificed for profit. Although this bit of wisdom has been denied over the years by investor-owned corporations, the practices of these corporations support the principle.

Several reports in the national press have demonstrated illegal, dishonest, and abusive practices associated with investor-owned hospital chains.[2] A large investor-owned hospital chain is under investigation by the FBI for escalating Medicare billing by falsifying Diagnostic Related Grouping (DRG) claims. The same corporation was convicted of violating labor laws to prevent nurses from unionizing. Other practices have been brought to light, such as limiting the stay after childbirth and persuading physicians to change DRGs. Most of the aberrations reported in the press arise from a desire to make profits on the part of administrators of the corporations or physicians who will send patients to the health care facilities operated by the corporations. Statistical studies demonstrate that investor-owned health maintenance organizations (HMOs) spend only 80 percent of their assets on patient care, whereas not-for-profit HMOs average more than 90 percent for patient care.[3] In sum, health care is a service, not a commodity; a profession, not a business.

In addition, some goods are so important for the well-being of people that they should be considered public goods—that is, goods that must be made available to all. Health care is one of those goods. This conviction does not result from religious teaching only; it was affirmed by a secular commission appointed by the federal government to study the health care system in the United States:

> Society has a moral obligation to ensure that everyone has access to adequate care without being subject to excessive burdens. . . . But the recognition of a collective or societal obligation does not imply that government should be the only or even the primary institution involved in the complex enterprise of making health care available. It is the Commission's view that the societal obligation to ensure

equitable access for everyone may best be fulfilled in this country by a pluralistic approach that relies upon the coordinated contributions of actions by both the private and public sectors.[4]

In the United States about 50 percent of the people have health care coverage by reason of employment. Others—for example, children with mothers who have limited income and people over age 65—have most of their health care costs funded by the federal government. Many people, however, fall in the cracks and do not have adequate access to health care. At present, this group totals forty million people. If persons are unable to achieve these goods, they should be provided by society. We recognize the importance of education, so we try to provide a basic education for all—including those who cannot afford to pay for it. To date, we have not considered health care to be of the same nature.

Although equal health care for all is not possible, basic care should be provided. To do this, we will probably have to change the manner in which we fund health care in the United States. In the past few years, many of the Medicaid patients previously cared for in city or county hospitals are now cared for in private hospitals. Does it seem unreasonable to suggest that the Medicaid program could be enlarged to care for those without adequate access at present?

Finally, other public goods include the education of health care professionals and research in health care. Both of these goods have been subsidized by health care fees in the past. With the effort to limit the costs of health care, however, less money will be available for these important public needs. Perhaps education and research should not be funded by fees for services as they have been in the past but from some other source. Other sources of public or private funds must be found to assure that these public goods will be provided in the future to the extent they have been in the past.

Conclusion

To some readers, the ideas presented here for a renewal of corporate health care in the United States are not surprising. They are foundational insofar as a just health care system is concerned. To others, the ideas proposed in this chapter might sound like a message from the Flat Earth Society. "How can anyone challenge the worth and validity of investor-owned health care corporations when they are so much in accord with the free enterprise economic system?" The argument presented here challenges the proponents of investor-owned health care corporations to demonstrate that overall, better patient care has resulted from market-driven activities or that our society benefits from a simple assumption that the market will solve all economic and health care needs and problems.

Notes

1. Jerome Kassirer, "Is Managed Care Here to Stay?" *New England Journal of Medicine* 336 (April 3, 1997):1014.
2. R. Pear, "U.S. Cites Criminals Raids on Medicare and Medicaid," *New York Times,* Nov. 4, 1999, A21.
3. George Church, "Backlash Against HMO's," *Time* (April 14, 1997), 32–36.
4. President's Commission for the Study of Ethical Problems in Medicine and Biomedical and Behavioral Research, *Securing Access to Health Care* (Washington, D.C.: Government Printing Office, 1983), 22–23.

Chapter 66 _____

Handling the 800-Pound Gorilla

As everyone knows, managed care has become the 800-pound gorilla dominating the American health care community. How does one handle an 800-pound gorilla? Very carefully! One interesting aspect of this phenomenon is that there are several descriptions of managed care. The most accurate description seems to come from John Iglehart: "Managed care seeks to reduce health care costs and improve quality of care by controlling choices traditionally made within the patient-physician relationship." Like any 800-pound gorilla, managed care has the reputation of being primarily destructive. Yet even a consistent critic of managed care admits, "The inherent virtues of managed care have manifested themselves in many salutary improvements to the system that might otherwise never have been made. Those include attempts to eliminate waste and redundancy, a greater focus on health promotion and disease prevention, more attention to the management of chronic diseases, a focus on the accountability of physicians and health plans on the quality of care, lower hospitalization rates without an obvious decline in the quality of care, heavy investment in patient information systems, and control of employer health care costs."[1]

Principles

In spite of these positive potentials, managed care plans have dark reputations in the minds of many patients and most physicians. A survey by a public relations firm of 589 citations in newspapers, magazines, and transcripts from television news programs found five unfavorable stories about managed care for every favorable story. In a national poll to rate industries in relation to service for consumers, managed care companies were ranked second from the bottom, above only tobacco companies. Managed care is associated with denial of care, gagging of physicians, callous treatment of women after childbirth and mastectomies, disproportionate attention to profits, refusal of emergency room care, and refusal to accept responsibility for medical teaching and research, to mention just a few complaints.

In an effort to dispel negative attitudes and limit the potential harm of managed care, two plans have been developed. The first, called Putting Patients First (PPF), was developed by the American Association of Health Plans (AAHP); it features a quality assessment program intended to detect any pattern of underservice, a clinical guideline program aimed at providing information and support for clinical decisions, a utilization-management program designed to evaluate the appropriateness of health care services, and a drug-formulating program aimed at informing physicians about pharmaco-economic information needed for cost effective medical practice. Under PPF, patients are to be informed of the various processes (such as utilization rules and drug formulary rules) only if they request such information. Compliance with the plan by AAHP members is voluntary. One commentator believes that the plan is worthless and is only "a thinly veiled attempt to ward off state and federal legislative actions to curb the abuse of managed care." A more friendly analysis of PPF is offered by David Jones, a board member of AAHP, who maintains that the plan "has teeth" and that it balances competing interests such as cost cutting, unlimited choice, and the practitioner's desire to be left alone.[2]

There probably will not be time to test the value and reliability of the PPF plan. Two other efforts under development to monitor and correct managed care might preempt PPF. The first, a Patient's Bill of Rights, was designed by a thirty-four-member presidential advisory committee. The committee suggested many of the same controls put forth in the PPF proposal but adds a stronger right of appeal. Decisions denying coverage could be appealed in court or to independent arbitrators. Many people have complained that enforcing all of the regulations in the Clinton plan would increase the cost of health care to the extent that managed care would lose its meaning.[3] The popular wisdom maintains that Republicans would be reluctant to listen to Clinton's appeals for enactment of the committee's proposal. They believe that regulation would stifle market forces that have reduced the cost of health care in the past three years.

Although the Patients' Bill of Rights might face the same fate as the 1992–93 effort to reform health care, Congress itself seems intent on enacting some limits upon managed care companies. Once again, however, Congress faces a delicate balance. If it responds too aggressively to the requests of constituents, it may impede the initiative and aggressive activities that led to the development of HMOs and other beneficial parts of the managed care movement.

Discussion

Although the various efforts to regulate managed care in the United States are significant, the question remains: Do they miss the mark? Will they tame the 800-pound gorilla? Three observations question the efficacy of the new regulations. First, the efforts of PPF, the Clinton committee, and the various proposed bills in Congress seem to have in mind the restoration of many premanaged care procedures. None of the new plans and proposed regulations mentions that the paradigm for health care has changed. In the past, health care was primarily concerned with doing everything possible for individual patients. Managed care, on the other hand, directs the attention of physicians and hospitals toward a group of patients, not only toward the patients who actively use the health care system. In the new paradigm, some of the new practices are reasonable, although they would have been rejected in the past. For example, a consistent practice of managed care allows patients access to specialists only after referral by a primary care physician. Seeking to mandate free access to specialists through law is anachronistic, yet this is the goal of several pieces of Congressional legislation.

Second, many of the standards put forth to measure the effectiveness of managed care programs are directed toward measuring customer satisfaction, not quality of care. Although customer satisfaction must be factored into an analysis of quality care, several other elements—such as outcome studies and information regarding competency of individual physicians and hospitals—also must be considered. It is much easier for a patient to express an opinion with regard to promptness in answering the phone (high on the list for patient satisfaction) than it is to measure the various outcomes for treating myocardial infarction. Yet the latter is a much more important factor in judging quality of care. Quality of care must be emphasized if progress is to be made in health care. Pre- and post-managed care medicine are both far from perfect. According to one observer, "One-fourth of hospital deaths may be preventable, and one-third of some hospital procedures may expose patients to risk without improving their health. One-third of drugs may not be indicated and one-third of tests showing abnormal results may not be followed up by physicians."[4]

Third, in the midst of forthcoming rules and regulations limiting the behavior of physicians and testing their commitments as well as their patience, perhaps physicians can cut the Gordian knot of increased regulations by putting into practice the words of an eminent pioneer in measuring quality of care: "I place the interactions of patients and practitioners at the center of the health care universe because I believe it is there that the processes and decisions most critical to quality take place. Here is the atomic furnace where quality is generated."[5] In other words, the profession of medicine achieves quality of care only if practitioners have empathy for their patients.

Conclusion

At the time of the Punic Wars, all sessions of the Roman Senate were concluded with the declaration, "Carthage must be destroyed". As a result of constant repetition this slogan became a goal of the Roman Republic, and it was eventually accomplished. With this in mind, it seems that when one reflects on managed care—its advantages and shortcomings—one is convinced that the only way to solve the health care problems in our society is to insist continually that we must have universal health care coverage. Until this goal is accomplished, we are fighting brush fires and ignoring the major conflagration.

Notes

1. J. Kassirer, "Is Managed Care Here to Stay?" *NEJM* 336 (April 3, 1997): 1014.
2. D. Jones, "Putting Patients First: A Philosophy in Practice," *Health Affairs* 16 (November/December 1997): 115–32.

3. P. Lee, "The True Test of Whether Health Plans Put Patients First," *Health Affairs* 16 (November/December 1997): 132–44.
4. R. Brook et al., "Health System Reform and Quality," *JAMA* 278 (August 14, 1996): 476.
5. A. Donabedian, "Quality in Health Care: Whose Responsibility Is It?" *American College of Medical Quality* (1993): 32.

Chapter 67 _____

The Oregon Health Care Plan: Some Questions

Several years ago in the state of Oregon, a seven-year-old boy died of leukemia. Shortly before his death, state health officials refused public funds for a potentially life-prolonging bone marrow transplant. In the same state, a young mother was refused public funding for a liver transplant. Both actions resulted from a new policy of state health officials to refuse funding for bone marrow, pancreas, heart, or liver transplants. The decisions in Oregon have been portrayed as a preview of decisions that will soon be necessary by officials in other states and by officials representing the federal government. Economic decisions that limit the access to health care have ethical implications. People will live or die as a result of these decisions. With this fact in mind, a closer investigation of the decisions in Oregon is in order.

Principles

Is there a general principle that will ensure an ethical distribution of public funds to people in need of health care? In Oregon, the painful decisions to withhold funds were based on the assumption that basic health care should be provided before advanced or experimental care. State officials in Oregon pointed out that basic health care was being provided for 24,000 more low-income people without any increase of funds by reason of the new policy. Moreover, they pointed out, 1,500 pregnant women will receive prenatal care with the same amount of money that would pay for thirty organ transplants.[1] Many commentators and editorial writers, applauding the wisdom and courage of the Oregon allotment policy, declared that Oregon should be a model for federal agencies faced with the same decisions. A consensus seemed to be present in the public forum that basic care for as many people as possible should be the principle upon which access to health care for lower-income people is determined.

The Oregon decisions occurred at a time when many people were searching for principles to regulate the amount of our national assets devoted to health care. In his provocative book *Setting Limits,* Daniel Callahan maintains that a new norm for funding health care for the aging must be developed.[2] At present, health care research and therapy in the United States seems to be directed toward keeping people alive as long as possible, no matter what degree of function they might retain. Callahan persuasively questions whether this norm is realistic, given the limited resources of our society and the certainty of death. He suggests that a more valid norm would be to afford as many people as possible the opportunity to live a beneficial life. Making such a radical readjustment in health care planning would direct funds away from the aging toward the younger members of society. Callahan realized that his idea is prophetic; he stated that it would not be accepted until his grandchildren are adults.

Discussion

The policies initiated in Oregon provide some guidance for the future. Moreover, Callahan's ideas (which are explained much more intelligently and compassionately in his book) must be considered as the issue of allotting funds for research and health care therapy is discussed. There is a vital question, however, that has not been considered sufficiently in Oregon or in Callahan's discussion: Are we a devoting fair share of national assets to health care for low-income people. Although we may posit that there are limited resources for health care, have we reached the reasonable limits of our resources? For the past twenty years, the proportion of our gross national product (GNP) devoted to health care has been a prominent discussion topic. A significant percentage of the GNP is devoted to items that can only be deemed ephermal. Are there many goods included in the GNP that are more important than access to health care? Moreover, it is that simple to distinguish between basic and advanced health care? If the criterion for distinguishing between basic and advanced health care is the success of the procedure, some types of organ transplant may be designated as basic care, and other types will soon be in that category.

A prominent health care economist pointed out in testimony before the Senate Commission on Aging that Americans are delighted when figures indicate that the automobile industry is flourishing because that "is good for the economy and good for the country." He asks whether the same attitude is not fitting insofar as health care is concerned. Without fostering a *laissez faire* attitude toward health care costs, we must admit Reinhardt is right in one regard: If we compare present and past percentages of the GNP devoted to health care, we are comparing apples and oranges. Though medicine still has the same goals it had forty years ago, the means and methods of reaching these goals have changed significantly.

Conclusion

According to the great Swiss theologian Karl Barth, a society must be judged on its willingness to care for its weak and impoverished members.[3] Although health care procedures should be carefully evaluated for cost efficiency, and although the function of a patient should be considered when evaluating the effectiveness of health care procedures, it seems equally important to evaluate whether our states and the federal government are devoting enough of our assets to offering access to health care for lower-income people.

Notes

1. Sana Rosenbaum, "Mothers and Children Last, The Oregon Medicaid Experiment," *American Journal of Law & Medicine,* XVII:142 (1992) 97–126.
2. Daniel Callahan, *Setting Limits, Medical Goals in an Aging Society.* (New York: Simon & Schuster, 1995).
3. Karl Barth, *Church Dogmatics,* (Grand Rapids, MI: Eerdmans, 1978).

Part Nine

Artificial Generation

Chapter 68 _____

In Vitro Fertilization and Surrogate Motherhood

When Arlette Schweitzer, forty-two years old, gave birth to twins in Aberdeen, South Dakota, it was not an unusual event, except for one factor: The twins were the result of *in vitro* fertilization (IVF) and embryo transplant, using ova from her daughter, Christa, and sperm from her son-in-law, Kevin Uchytil. In other words, through the assistance of technicians and technology, Arlette Schweitzer became the "mother" of her genetic grandchildren. Although a woman in South Africa played the same role in the generation of triplets in 1987, the South Dakota case was the first of its kind in the United States. Once again, this process of fertilization, gestation, and birth prompted an evaluation of *in vitro* fertilization and surrogate "motherhood" in general and the Schweitzer-Uchytil collaboration in particular. This chapter recounts some of the discussion and seeks to contribute to the discussion from an ethical perspective. In addition to presenting a unique family situation, the case offers a fascinating example of the way different ethical methods are utilized in the United States, as well as the varying results of these different methods.

Principles

Most people commenting upon the Schweitzer-Uchytil collaboration focused exclusively on the ultimate intentions of the persons involved. This form of ethical evaluation is most popular in the United States. If the facts and the outcome of the Schweitzer-Uchytil case are evaluated from the viewpoint of intention, the action would be "good." Two young married persons wish to have a child, but because the mother was born without a uterus they are unable to generate children through the natural process of sexual intercourse. By means of IVF and transplant of the zygote into the womb of Christa's mother, they are able to use their own genetic material to cooperate in the production of new persons. Arlette Schweitzer stated that carrying the babies "was an act of love; I never had any second thoughts." Hence, the ultimate intentions of all parties seem to be above reproach.

The problem with evaluating human actions solely from the viewpoint of the ultimate intention is that almost any action or group of actions joined together by an ultimate intention might be evaluated as "good" if the intention is good. In the 1950s an academic type defended the actions of Adolph Hitler because the ultimate intention of all of his actions was "the good of the Fatherland." Without questioning the ultimate intentions of the people involved in the Schweitzer-Uchytil case, a more thorough ethical analysis is needed. The impact on the overall well-being of all persons involved in the series of actions that produced the desired effect should be analyzed. The term "overall well-being" implies that we must evaluate the effect of the free human acts on the functions or capacities of the persons involved—that is, the physical, psychological, social, and creative (spiritual) capacities of the persons.

Probing the effects of actions on the physical, psychological, social, and creative functions or capacities of the person is not always easy. Because these human functions or capacities exist in the unity of a person, the effect on the capacities or functions of the person should not be analyzed disjunctively but in an integrated manner. The aforementioned functions of the human personality are related as dimensions of a cube, not as layers in a cake. Although a layer of cake may be removed and the remains would still be a cake, if a dimension of a cube is removed the cube ceases to be. Though one function may be more important than another—for example, the creative function is considered the most important because to some extent it is directive of the others—no function can be sacrificed for another. Could we think and love (creative functions) without our bodies? Our physiological function, though in some ways the least "dignified" level of human function, must not be manipulated or sacrificed except for the good of the whole body. For this reason, we consider the removal of diseased organs to save the whole body a good action. We do not approve, however, of mutilating our bodies for money (social good). Thus, we consider selling the organs of a living person, such as a kidney, as unethical. We are not persons (spirits) merely existing in bodies; we are persons because we have bodies. As persons, we are an integrated unity of body and spirit.

Discussion

Does this method of ethical evaluation help us in evaluating the case in question? The principal persons involved in IVF using genetic material supplied by a married couple, later completed by embryo transplant, are the wife and husband, the woman who serves as surrogate, and the children resulting if the process is successful. Let us briefly consider the effect on these people.

The husband and wife who supply the genetic material for the new children may impose unforeseen burdens on themselves. Paul Lauritzen, speaking for himself and his wife, sums up the experience of their efforts to generate children through technological processes by saying, "The process of reproduction in a clinical environment (causes) a way of thinking of ourselves and our world in terms that are incompatible with intimacy. . . . Once procreation is separated from sexual intercourse, it is difficult not to treat the process of procreation as the production of an object to which one has the right as a producer. It is also difficult under these circumstances to place the end above the means: Effectiveness in accomplishing one's goal can easily become the sole criterion by which decisions are made.[1]

Nature (evolution) has designed the act of generation (sexual intercourse) as a fully human act; it involves all the functions of the persons who come together to perform the action. Moreover, it requires and enhances intimacy between two people. As a result of this intimacy, the couple willingly gestate, nurture, and educate the embryo, infant, child. If intimacy is lacking, as the Lauritzens avow, will generation through IVF and surrogate gestation be beneficial for parents and child? The objection to IVF may be phrased this way: Will IVF result in the deprivation of some vital familial goods that loving intercourse provides? When IVF is used in the process of fertilization of genetic material, the child that results is not generated in a human fashion; it is manufactured. Will this fact make a difference? Is it possible to inflict harm on ourselves and others by circumventing or ignoring the process of nature? We have seen the damage we have done to our environment by ignoring nature. Are we setting ourselves up for the same type of disaster by ignoring the ecology of human generation? Finally, as another drawback of assisted reproduction, Lauritzen maintains, "The cycle of hope and then despair that repeats itself in unsuccessful fertility treatments can become unbearable."

With regard to the gestational mother, who is to nurture the fetuses for nine months and then give them up, a serious psychological, social, and creative burden also may be imposed on her. As the Baby M case indicated, surrogate motherhood demands that the woman who is the gestational mother not act like a mother. The bonding that occurs between a mother and infant in the womb is stronger and more long-lasting than any other human bond. Is it beneficial or even possible for a woman to act like a mother for nine months and then sever the deepest human ties and pretend she is not the mother of her child for the rest of her life?

The children of IVF and surrogate gestation may also be deprived in the process. A sense of identity needed for healthy personal development is founded on the knowledge that one knows one's parents. The development of identity in each person results from gestation. nurturing, and education. These three elements are a continuum. Will separating the elements of this process injure children? Will IVF and gestational surrogacy weaken family bonds as children grow older and wonder about their "real" parents?

Conclusion

Coping with infertility is a difficult burden for married people. Clearly, some methods of coping with this burden will be more beneficial than others. Coping through IVF and embryo transplant to a surrogate mother may not be as problem-free a method of coping as once believed.

Note

1. Paul Lauritzen, "What Price Parenthood?" *Hastings Center Report* 20 (March/April 1990), 38–46.

Chapter 69 _____

Conceiving One Child to Save Another

Abe and Mary Ayala, a California couple in their mid-forties, did not plan to have another child. They changed their minds, however, when their seventeen-year-old daughter, Anissa, was diagnosed with leukemia—a cancer of the blood cells that can sometimes be cured by transplanting bone marrow cells from a compatible donor. Because the medical team could not find a suitable donor among relatives or friends, the Ayalas decided to have another child, taking a one-in-four chance that the newborn child would be a compatible bone marrow donor for Anissa. The gamble seems to be paying off: Prenatal testing indicates that the female fetus will be a compatible bone marrow donor.

When the Ayala story became public, medical ethicists were consulted, and some criticized the venture because the newly conceived child was being treated as a "means," not as an "end." In response to the observations of the ethicists, several media persons affirmed the right of the Ayalas to do whatever they desired as long as love is their motive. At the same time, some columnists berated the ethicists for offering opinions from an ivory tower. Can we evaluate the actions of the Ayalas from an ethical perspective? Does ethics have anything to offer with regard to such a personal and emotion-laden decision?

Principles

Although no method of ethical evaluation eliminates emotional reactions, there are distinctions and considerations that may help to minimize them. First, it is necessary to distinguish the remote intention or purpose of the act in question from the intention or purpose embodied in the act itself. If the remote intention of an action is emphasized to the exclusion of the proximate intention expressed in the act itself, one can justify just about anything. If I rob poor widows to pay for my college education and consider only the remote intention, then robbing widows might be put forth as a good action because it enabled me to obtain a college education. Discussions concerning the morality of abortion often break down because of the failure to make this distinction. In the case of the Ayalas, their desire to prolong the life of Anissa is a good intention. The means they utilize to prolong her life must be evaluated in their own right, however. Is it ethically acceptable to conceive a child mainly with the intention of providing therapy for another child? That is the ethical issue under consideration.

In assessing an action with emotional overtones, it is helpful to step back and ask, "What if everybody performed the action with the same purpose in mind?" Immanuel Kant recommended that a similar question be asked in forming ethical norms: What if every child were conceived as a means to prolong the life of other living persons? What would this situation do to our society and to the self-esteem of children as they progress to maturity?

Another approach that helps us to evaluate an emotion-laden action is to consider the action from a perspective that everyone would consider acceptable. Then we can consider the action in question from a perspective that all would consider perverse. Finally, we can compare the action in question to good and perverse actions to determine whether it more closely resembles the good action or the perverse action. For example, if a child is conceived as a sign and result of the mutual love of the parents and is nurtured and educated with the intention of helping the child attain human fulfillment, most people would agree that conceiving the child is a good action. On the other hand, everyone would agree that conceiving children to sell them into slavery would be wrong because it debases and devalues the worth and dignity of the human persons who will be slaves. Even if the parents plead poverty and state that their children will have a more comfortable life in slavery than if they were to stay with their poor parents, the act of generating human beings with the intention of selling them into slavery is simply unacceptable. A child should never be considered the property of the parents. Clearly, generating a child as a potential bone marrow donor is not exactly the same as conceiving a child to sell him or her into slavery. Does the intention of the Ayalas resemble more closely the good or the perverse intention?

Discussion

Mrs. Ayala responded to the remarks of ethicists by saying, "We are going to love our baby. Our baby is going to have more love than she probably can put up with." Without questioning the Ayalas' overall dispositions, Mrs. Ayala's statement illustrates the difficulty of accurately using the word "love" in the English language. In English, we convey three different human actions through the word "love." In Greek three words are used to convey these three types of love: *philia, eros,* and *agape.* The significance of this examination of words and concepts is that the deepest form of human love, *agape,* is the type of love we predicate between parents and children. *Agape* is incompatible with self-serving intentions. Can we say we have the deepest form of love for another (*agape*) if we are going to use that other person to achieve goals that we have determined without consulting the person in question? Thus, the need for more accurate distinctions and soul-searching evaluation when we use the word "love" to justify human actions.

Stepping back from the immediate question once more, consider the activity and outlook of the physicians who advised the Ayalas. Although they remained behind the scenes insofar as the news stories were concerned, they probably were deeply involved in the decision to create a "suitable" bone marrow donor. Once again, we face the question: Is the goal of medicine to prolong life as long as possible, no matter what means are used? Or is the goal of medicine to help people pursue a better life, the worth and dignity of all persons being respected in the process? If one opts for prolonging life as the ultimate purpose of medical care, the patient (and/or family) is often subjected to therapy with no regard for the values and priorities of the person. Most cases of overtreatment as death approaches are examples of the "prolonging life at all costs" outlook. In the immediate future, as our ability to prolong life increases—for example, through mechanical devices such as the artificial heart or through xenografts—the question of human benefit must be put in the forefront of medical and ethical decisions. What risks and burdens are to be endured to prolong one's own life or the life of another?

Conclusion

Finally, do ethicists have any role in commenting on personal and emotion-laden decisions that have ethical ramifications? Seemingly, they have as much right to comment as do newspaper columnists, but this observation doesn't answer the question. Clearly, the observations of ethicists are offered more effectively before than after the fact. If offered after the fact, the observations must be thorough and circumspect, or they will be lost in the emotional reaction to which they give rise.

Part Ten

❖

Special Questions

Chapter 70 _____

On Playing God

Consider the situation: Health care professionals appear on a radio or TV talk show devoted to questions concerning the treatment of severely debilitated patients. If the proposed ethical solution suggests that a person be allowed to die, someone will object to the solution and say, "You are playing God." This phrase is usually uttered with the implied meaning, "Life-and-death decisions in medical care must be left to God. Human beings have no right to interfere with God's work." Is this attitude reasonable? Is there any sense in which human beings can and should "play God"? Or should human beings be more cautious, withdrawing from decision making when it becomes obvious that death might unavoidably ensue if another good is chosen? Understanding the concept of "playing God" will help us understand better the mission, nobility, and limits of medicine.

Principles

The term *God* implies an all-powerful, wise, and good being whom human beings worship as creator and ruler of the universe. God is the provident director of events and happenings in the universe. Persons who do not believe in a personal God might substitute for God the term *nature*, meaning "a creative and controlling force in the universe."

Is there any sense in which human beings ought to "play God" or "assume the role of nature"? The glory and challenge of being human is that we are called on to "play God": We are challenged to assist nature by being creative and by controlling our own lives and the happenings of the environment. If we are to fulfill our humanity, we must take an active role in shaping our own destiny, help others fulfill their destiny, and maintain the ecology of the universe. We are created in the image and likeness of God. We have powers from God (nature)—our intellect and our will—that enable us to take an active and determining role in the decisions affecting our lives and our destinies. We can respect and develop our person and capacities, whether mental or physical, or allow them to deteriorate and atrophy. We can build great societies or allow ourselves to destroy one another through bitterness, envy, and violence. We can respect our environment and preserve it for generations to come, or we can ravage it rapaciously and leave a wasteland for our progeny.

Medical research is an illustrative example of our ability and need to "play God." Medical research seeks to improve human life by eliminating disease and improving our quality of life. Would it be fitting for the medical community to remain passive in the face of the AIDS epidemic and say, "This is God's way of punishing people and we must not interfere"? Of course not. The medical research community, at the behest of all caring people, plays God and tries to eliminate AIDS, thus controlling the future and eventually eliminating one more source of human suffering.

In medical matters, most people realize the need to be responsible for personal health. Realizing that they cannot expect God to send medical care unless they do something about seeking out this help, most people will seek medical help if they are ill. Few people realize, however, that we have the power and responsibility to be creative and controlling with regard to other facets of medical care. By working together we can provide more adequate health care for all members of our society. Moreover, through mutual cooperation we can improve our environment and the quality of life in our cities.

Although we have the power to "play God" or influence nature regarding our personal, social, and ecological responsibilities, we do not have unlimited power. God has unlimited power, but humans are limited. Unfortunately, admitting limitations and shortcomings seems to be difficult for human beings. If we choose one goal, it usually means we must relinquish another. By choosing to avoid physical or mental suffering, a person with a fatal pathology may also reject life-prolonging therapy and thus hasten death. We cannot have it all. "Playing God" in the sense of not admitting limitations leads ultimately to personal unhappiness and social disaster. Thus, we are called on to "play God" insofar as being creative and planning for the future is concerned. To realize this power responsibly, however, we must recognize our limitations.

Discussion

Medical professionals tend to ignore subconsciously the limitations of knowledge and technique. Some physicians, for example, act as though the death of a patient is a personal defeat. Thus, physicians themselves testify that patients who have incurable and terminal disease often are not given the same attention as those who may recover from their illness. Given the limitations of human beings, helping people die well is just as much a part of medical care as healing. Knowing when to cure and when to simply care is the epitome of the science and art of medicine.

Admitting limitations for research programs is also difficult. Do people who set policy for research programs stop to ask, "We can't do everything; what are the most beneficial things we can do with our limited resources?" Instead, political and economic pressures seem to determine the research agenda. In the United States, medical care and research programs emphasize experimental procedures such as transplants and artificial organs for the few, whereas more basic programs for the many—such as neonatal care—often are neglected. Although medical progress requires that some attention be given to experimental procedures, are policies on research and practice formulated with a view to social as well as personal medical needs? A neutral observer evaluating U.S. research programs' medical practice might conclude that these programs are based on the assumptions that medical care can enable people to live forever and that there are unlimited financial resources.

Besides health care professionals, the general public also often presumes that no limitations exist to health care funding. Many people see an egregious violation of human rights if a representative of a health care facility—especially a Catholic facility—is forced to say, "I am sorry, we don't have the funds to accept you as a patient." True, health care institutions (especially Catholic ones), by reason of the profession to which they are dedicated, should do as much charity care as possible. Institutions as well as individual persons have limits, however, and facilities that publicly acknowledge these limits do not violate others' rights.

Conclusion

"Playing God" in a worthwhile sense means that we realize we are responsible for the destiny of ourselves, others, and the environment. It also means that in fulfilling our responsibilities we must admit our limitations. Admitting limitations is simply another way of saying that we must pose relevant ethical questions.

Chapter 71 _____

Autopsy: Ethical and Religious Considerations

At times, people are reluctant to release the body of a loved one for autopsy. Are there good reasons for this reluctance? Is it a violation of propriety, ethics, or religion to release the body of a spouse, parent, or child for medical examination? If not, why the continued reluctance?

Principles

When a human being dies, the body is no longer unified by the life-giving principle or soul by which it is a constituted human being. The cadaver of a person, then, is not a *human* body in the proper sense of the word. Insofar as possible, we should avoid referring to the physical remains of a person as though the person existed *in* a human body or was, so to speak, limited by the human body. Although existing in this life, the human person is a substantial unity of spirit (form) and body (matter), not an accidental juxtaposition of two distinct entities. Although the remains of a human body may resemble the body of a living person, and although this resemblance may be prolonged through embalming, the remains are not a human body but a mass of organic matter, decomposing into constitutive organic elements.

If the corpse of a human person is not a human body, why are people so concerned about proper care for the remains of the deceased person? Why treat it with the respect and reverence it usually receives? Respect and reverence are owed to the remains of a human being because of the value of human life that once informed the now inert mass still bearing the image of the deceased person. To mourn and express sorrow for the fact that the person will no longer be present in the same manner as before, the people who remain perform certain reverential actions that express their love. Respect for the dead body, then, signifies respect for human life, respect for God, and respect for the person who once subsisted with this now corrupting corpse and who now exists in a different modality. Hence, the actions and rituals that people follow when caring for the body of a deceased person have a meaning beyond their apparent signification.

Autopsy is the examination of a cadaver after death, performed to provide greater medical knowledge concerning the cause of death. Historically, the first major impetus for autopsies was provided when Frederick II, emperor of the Holy Roman Empire, instructed physicians studying at Salerno and Naples to spend at least one year in the study of anatomy. Theologians expressed the belief that such dissection of the human cadaver could be done with proper respect for the dead as long as the organs were restored to the body before burial.

In accord with the respect due the remains of a human being, then, in an autopsy no organ should be removed from a corpse, nor should the body be dismembered in any way, unless there is a sufficient reason to justify such an action. Usually the next-of-kin or the person to whom the corpse is committed for care has the legal right to determine if organs may be removed from the body and if an autopsy may be performed (*Pierce v. Swan Point,* 1872). The right of the next-of-kin with regard to caring for the human body is not absolute, however. It may be superseded by statements made by the person while still alive—such as a wish to donate his or her body for scientific study—or by the needs of society, such as when an autopsy might help improve medical knowledge.

An autopsy occasionally will provide knowledge about a rare or contagious disease. In such cases, autopsies should be performed because the good of the community demands it and because increased medical knowledge is needed. If the next-of-kin were not willing to approve the autopsy, the court could order that the autopsy be performed. In cases of violent death or unattended death, an autopsy is required by law, no matter what wishes are expressed by the next of kin.

Usually, however, the purpose of an autopsy is not to trace the etiology of a rare disease or to discover unknown or violent causes of death. More frequently, autopsies are performed to help health care professionals achieve a higher level of effectiveness in the care of the living. Autopsies are especially useful for the common good when they are performed in teaching hospitals. The autopsy rate of a hospital is usually a sign of concern for excellence; it offers a gauge of professional integrity and interest in scientific advancement. Through autopsies, the diagnosis and treatment a person received can be evaluated and staff members encouraged to observe a high level of proficiency.

Discussion

From a Christian point of view, the practice of allowing autopsies on one's body for scientific research is acceptable and even to be encouraged if a true need exists. Pope Pius XII, for example, exhibited approval of autopsies when he said,

> The public must be educated. It must be explained with intelligence
> and respect that to consent explicitly or tacitly to serious damage to
> the integrity of the corpse in the interest of those who are suffering,
> is no violation of the reverence due to the dead.[1]

According to the prevailing opinion of Jewish scholars, autopsies can be condoned only when there are indications that the information accruing from them may be of value in saving the life of another individual. Thus, postmortem dissections are indicated when an experimental drug or surgical procedure was used and the autopsy is likely to shed some light on the merits of the treatment. Similarly, when death was caused by contagious disease or genetic disorder, autopsies are warranted for the purpose of instituting prophylactic treatment or helping with genetic counseling for others. Most rabbinic authorities also permit postmortem dissection for forensic purposes when mandated by law. In all cases where autopsies are indicated, they must be limited to the special areas where relevant information may be obtained. After the examination, all organs must be returned for burial.

The teaching of Islam does not allow for voluntary autopsy because it is considered a desecration of the human person who was associated with the body. If the law requires it, however, the next-of-kin may acquiesce to it. Unless some law would be broken or public health endangered, the religious beliefs of people who disapprove of autopsies should be respected. It is worthwhile to point out, however, that one reason why medicine in the Islamic world failed to progress after a promising beginning was because of a lack of clinical information that could have been garnered through autopsies.

Because of what a corpse represents, it should be shown respect and reverence. Such respect and reverence is consistent with autopsies that are designed to promote public health and improve medical knowledge, provided proper respect is shown for the cadavers. When people are faced with a decision concerning autopsy, they should be encouraged to approve such a procedure because of the help that will be offered to others.

Note

1. Pope Pius XII, *The Human Body* (Boston: St. Paul Press, 1960), 382.

Chapter 72 _____

Pain: Some Ethical Considerations

Pain is a continual concern of the human community. Indeed, one can envision pain, in one form or another, as the *raison d'etre* of all professions. Pain may arise from many sources: spiritual, social, emotional, or physiological. For health care professionals, pain is described as "an unpleasant sensory or emotional experience associated with actual or potential tissue damage or described in terms of such damage"[1]. At one time, pain was considered an unwanted but necessary by-product of disease and illness. Terminal cancer patients, for example, would usually experience severe pain as death approached. In recent years, however, significant progress has been made in the control of pain. This chapter is interested not in pain as a medical reality but in pain and pain control as they present ethical concerns. Thus, here we consider the meaning of pain and the ethical response to pain on the part of health care professionals.

The Meaning of Pain

For the most part, health care professionals and patients alike avoid the question: Why pain? A few considerations garnered from the wisdom of experience and religious tradition may help to put pain in better perspective, however. The term *pain* is derived from the Latin term *poena,* which means penalty. Unfortunately, as the book of Job attests, many people take the term *poena* literally and consider illness, disease, and the pain that accompanies them as a penalty for evil behavior. Thus, pain becomes for many people a sign of God's displeasure and a punishment for moral faults. If this were true, however, only evil persons would suffer—and we know that is not the case. Although some religious traditions do trace the presence of evil and pain in the world to a general shortcoming of the whole human race, they do not present it as part of God's original plan or as a punishment for personal sin.

Having said what pain is not, can we say anything about the meaning of pain? To question the meaning of pain is to question the meaning of all evil—even death. The problem of pain and evil is a Gordian knot that all great religious traditions seek to unravel. How could an all-merciful God allow pain and suffering to exist in the world? How could a loving God allow a young child to suffer from the pain of leukemia or the generous mother of five to die in pain when others, dedicated to their own pleasures, are left untouched? The depth of this question about a loving God and the suffering of the innocent has turned many people to agnosticism.

People of faith realize that questions of pain and suffering will always be a mystery. Although people of faith perceive God as provident and loving, they do not know God as God knows himself and so cannot understand why God allows pain and suffering. To say that pain and suffering are a mystery is simply an admission that human beings are dependent on God and cannot know everything. In the Christian tradition, pain and suffering have been considered an opportunity for the individual to join his or her suffering to that of Jesus and thus dispose for greater spiritual union with God. Most world religions envision some form of transforming experience through the proper acceptance of pain and suffering.

Because of the effort to transform pain and suffering, critics have considered Christianity and other world religions masochistic. Accepting pain and suffering as a necessary component of human life, however, is not the same as saying that pain and suffering are good or that they are desired by God. Hence, world religions have always considered the conquering and alleviation of pain and suffering as a fundamental responsibility of the human community.

Discussion

What is the ethical response to pain for health care professionals? When a patient is in pain, the health care professional has three ethical responsibilities: to recognize the effect that the pain and suffering of patients will have on the health care professional; to help the patient transform the pain into a beneficial experience; and to alleviate or remove the pain if possible.

A seldom-realized phenomenon is the detrimental effect that living with the pain and suffering of patients may have on health care professionals. Sound understanding of human personality helps us realize that people who live in the presence of pain will be affected by it. If one does not have a beneficial method of dispelling the sorrow of pain and suffering, one becomes insensitive to the suffering of others.

Although suffering should never be sought for its own sake, at times it cannot be avoided. In these circumstances, it may become a source of spiritual growth. Helping patients use their fear and suffering as a transforming experience requires personal involvement on the part of the health care professional. Faced with a suffering and dying patient, some health care professionals turn the patient over to the pastoral care team and remain very much in the background. Others see the care of suffering and dying patients as a mutual responsibility with pastoral care persons. Pediatricians seem to consider it part of their responsibility to help children die in peace.

Alleviating and eliminating pain is much more possible today than in the past. As in any other medical procedure, the patient or proxy should be consulted with regard to the use of devices to control pain. Many methods to relieve pain or alleviate suffering result in reduced awareness or consciousness in the patient. Some people would rather experience manageable pain than lose their power of concentration. Moreover, different persons have different thresholds of pain. Assigning the same therapy for all persons in pain therefore is not an ethical procedure.

At times, the need to alleviate pain may require the use of analgesics that indirectly shorten life. In such circumstances, this is an act of mercy designed to relieve pain, not an act of euthanasia designed to kill the person. Although the side effect of this act of mercy may be to hasten death, the side effect is unintended. For example, a person who is removed from a respirator because life-sustaining efforts are unsuccessful will experience dyspnea or severe discomfort. In this case, morphine sulphate or other barbiturate may be administered to alleviate the pain, even if death is hastened. Utilizing morphine before determining the actual pain of the patient has been criticized as causing death rather than relieving pain. Patients removed from ventilators follow a predictable pattern involving pain, however, and this pattern can be reasonably predicted.[2] Thus, using morphine before the patient is removed from the ventilator would seem to be an ethical practice.

Notes

1. Institute for the Study of Pain, 1994.
2. L. Scheiderman and R. Sprag, "Ethical Decisions in Discontinuing Mechanical Ventilation," *NEJM.* vol 318 (April 15, 1988), 984–89.

Chapter 73

Suffering and the Need for Compassion

A few years ago, Janet Adkins was diagnosed as being in the early stages of Alzheimer's disease. Less than a year later, she killed herself, using a "suicide machine" invented and offered for use by retired physician Jack Kevorkian. In defending his involvement in the case, Kevorkian argued that, in light of the circumstances in which Mrs. Adkins found herself, his assistance in her self-induced death was the only appropriate thing to do. Responses from the medical profession, ethicists, and others were swift and fairly uniform in their condemnation of Kevorkian's actions. Citing the Hippocratic oath—which counsels physicians to "neither give a deadly drug to anybody . . . nor to make a suggestion to this effect"—critics expressed concern about the erosion of trust in the medical profession that such action could cause. Although this concern is legitimate, it does not get to the heart of the matter.

More to the point, Janet Adkins was suffering not physically but psychically. She looked ahead to a life of increasing disability and dependence and found these possibilities inconsistent with her view of meaningful life. She went to a physician for help in managing the reality she faced. The physician did what many others do when presented with this kind of situation: He turned to technology for a "quick fix."

The Limits of Technology

As a society, we are becoming increasingly and painfully aware that medical knowledge and technology often cannot provide relief for suffering, particularly suffering of the kind Mrs. Adkins had. As a result, physicians—who are accustomed to relying on scientific knowledge and technical expertise to exercise power and control over illness—may at times such as these experience powerlessness and, as a result, a sense of personal vulnerability. What is called for by way of response is neither the inappropriate application of technology nor the simple quoting of oaths in an attempt to justify passivity, inaction, or withdrawal. A fitting response to suffering demands at least two things of physicians. First, physicians must understand the nature and meaning of suffering as distinct from pain—whether physical, emotional, or spiritual. Second, they must understand that when science and technology have little to offer in response to suffering, the physician still is called upon to be compassionate.

The Nature and Meaning of Suffering

Although suffering may be concomitant with pain, it is not the same as pain. Suffering is a more profound experience wherein the integrity and meaning of the self are threatened. The person who suffers is tormented by fear, not only fear of the possibility of physical discomfort or loss of life, but fear of loss of self and self-identity. For example, when a person is told that he or she has Alzheimer's disease, that person's first thoughts may be about future isolation from loved ones and friends that can occur because of memory loss or confusion. Often, the suffering person initially retreats into a world of silence in an attempt to "make sense" of the painful reality that threatens, whether that reality is a disturbing diagnosis, the recent loss of a loved one, or a reversal in the fortunes of life. If the person is to manage the initial threat to self and emerge psychically intact from this period of silence, he or she must find words to express, and thereby gain some control over, what is being experienced. The search for words and language has twofold importance. First, it provides an opportunity for the person to look with a degree of objectivity at the events in the past that threaten the integrity of the self—for example, receiving the diagnosis of Alzheimer's disease. Second, it allows the person to project into the future a new self, reconstituted in light of the devastating reality that brings on the experience of suffering.

Once the person finds a voice to express the pain and fear associated with the experience, there then exists the possibility for hope in the future—albeit a different future than the one originally anticipated. This process entails a transformation wherein the suffering is not eliminated but is made manageable and a new sense of meaning and self-identity can emerge.

Technology and scientific expertise offer little help in addressing suffering of this kind. As a result, the physician may have a tendency to refer the suffering patient to a counselor, psychiatrist, or chaplain. The physician's responsibility to the patient does not end at the limits of medicine and technology, however, nor does the physician's "power" in the healing relationship. Perhaps more than at any other time in the experience of illness, the person who suffers this kind of threat to the self needs to be empowered if healing is to be effected. Empowerment of this kind is possible only through compassionate presence and response to the person who suffers.

The Compassionate Physician

Unfortunately, the scientific practice of medicine can act as a strong deterrent to compassionate response. Insofar as medicine's focus is pathophysiology, suffering can escape its glance. More important, however, medicine's emphasis on deductive science and its suspicion that the subjective element can distract the clinician from scientific data can lead to the "don't get too involved with your patient or you'll burn out" syndrome.

True compassion, however, demands what the highly deductive and objective approach finds suspect. The compassionate physician is willing to enter into a process with the suffering person and offer help in accepting and moving beyond the reality that poses the destructive threat to the self. This kind of response requires of the physician a degree of identification with the patient that is likely to increase the physician's own vulnerability in the encounter. Unless the physician has a genuine openness and vulnerability, however, the sufferer is unlikely to experience the encounter as a healing one in the fullest sense.

Movement through the states of suffering from silent fear to hope in a new future is facilitated by the presence of a compassionate other. The physician who is willing to enter this process with a suffering person not only affirms in word and deed who the person is in the present but also affirms and accepts who the person will be in the future.

Of course, no conclusions can be drawn about what Janet Adkins would have done had the physician she went to for help offered her at least the opportunity to search for hope for the future rather than closing off the future with one stroke of technology. One thing is certain: No "salvation" or solutions to the human problems encountered in suffering are offered by narrow reliance on scientific and technological expertise. Empowerment of the one who suffers, and thereby true healing, is effected only by the response of compassionate people.

Chapter 74 _____

Truth-Telling and Alzheimer's Disease

In the early 1960s, studies indicated that a majority of physicians would withhold a diagnosis of terminal cancer from their patients. Physicians cited fears of adverse reactions by patients to information and the destruction of patient hopes as reasons for withholding a diagnosis. By the late 1970s, similar studies demonstrated a radical shift in physician practice: More than 95 percent of doctors told their patients of the cancer diagnosis. The shift in emphasis in the physician-patient relationship from paternalism to autonomy has led many physicians to disclose the full truth of diagnosis to their patients. Recent literature has examined similar truth-telling questions about Huntington's disease and multiple sclerosis and reached conclusions consistent with that new model of disclosure. Today, more complicated questions arise. What information should be revealed to a patient with an Alzheimer's type disease? Can a case be made for withholding a diagnosis from such a patient? If so, under what conditions should that be done?

Principles

Often, people analyze ethical responsibilities on the basis of normative principles such as autonomy, beneficence, confidentiality, and honesty. Yet these principles may conflict with each other (e.g., autonomy versus non-maleficence). Thus, a more helpful method of ethical decision making considers the patient's ability to achieve human fulfillment through the integration of physiological, psychological, social, and creative goods.

In this context the patient has a responsibility to seek health because it is a basic human good. To exercise this responsibility, the patient must have sufficient information to make an informed decision about medical treatment in light of personal values. Because the physician-patient relationship involves mutual responsibilities, the patient and the physician have the respective duties to seek out and provide information that will promote responsible treatment choices and life decisions that are consistent with the patient's effort to seek true human fulfillment. To achieve this goal, the physician provides information that is truthful, useful, and has the capacity to help patients make reasonable decisions.

First and foremost, the information must be truthful because trust remains at the heart of the physician-patient relationship. Deception and failure to disclose information will undermine such trust. Second, physicians constantly make determinations about what information is useful, often excluding esoteric medical facts from the sharing process. Ordinarily, *useful* information is information that which a "reasonable" person would desire. Such a standard for disclosure must be tempered, however, by individual patient needs. The information provided should enable patients to understand adequately their condition and make informed decisions. Third, the information need only provide the capacity to promote patient good. The fact that the information may cause adverse effects (e.g., depression, anxiety, or even suicidal thoughts) should not dissuade the physician from revealing pertinent diagnostic or prognostic information. In fact, physicians frequently offer treatments (surgeries, chemotherapies, etc.) that have potential adverse effects; they offer such treatments if they provide some potential to help the patient strive for integral human fulfillment. If a physician suspects strongly that the information may cause serious and immediate adverse effects, however, disclosure may be delayed temporarily until appropriate support systems are arranged to help the patient deal with the truth. This delay involves a particular application of therapeutic privilege wherein less than full disclosure is appropriate to avoid countertherapeutic results. Finally, if the sharing of information has no capacity to help patients strive after their purpose in life, disclosure is not mandated. This scenario is analogous to a physician not being required to offer a "futile" medical treatment.

Studies support the need for truth-telling. Patients with actual diseases and others when presented with a hypothetical diagnosis indicate a desire to know the truth about the diagnosis. Granted, the information may be upsetting for patients at first, but there is no good documentation of the harmful consequences that truth-telling allegedly engenders. Provision of information allows patients to make informed decisions for further treatment and to prepare for the future. In addition, such information relieves patient anxiety caused by a fear of the unknown. Furthermore, disclosure avoids embarrassment when the patient inadvertently discovers withheld information. Finally, by naming a disease, the patient often gains symbolic control over it.

In sum, patients should be told the truth not merely for the sake of fulfilling an abstract principle of truth-telling. The truth is told in the context of concern and compassion, to promote true human fulfillment. The temporary exception to full disclosure (i.e., the application of therapeutic privilege) must be scrutinized carefully with a view toward creating a situation in which full disclosure ultimately can occur.

Discussion

Like the word "cancer" years ago, today the word "Alzheimer's" strikes terror in the minds of patients and families. Such terror motivated Janet Adkins to commit suicide with the aid of Dr. Jack Kevorkian. Do such cases suggest that information about an Alzheimer's diagnosis be withheld from the patient?

An application of the principles regarding truth-telling outlined above produces a *prima facie* presumption for full disclosure to the Alzheimer's patient. Additional factors must be considered, however. First, no cure presently exists for Alzheimer's disease, although there is a growing battery of symptomatic relief. Second, definite diagnosis of the disease occurs only upon histopathologic confirmation after autopsy. Laboratory, clinical, and imaging tests provide only probable diagnosis, allowing for possible misdiagnosis. Third, an Alzheimer's patient often lacks the capacity to make decisions because he or she is unable to retain and process information.

Nevertheless, such additional factors do not seem to modify greatly the responsibility to disclose a diagnosis. First, the lack of a cure does not make Alzheimer's unique. Many diseases are incurable, yet disclosure is made. Withholding tragic or terminal diagnoses may subvert the nature of medicine by giving the impression that the sole purpose of medicine is to cure. In reality, sometimes medicine cannot cure. The fact that on rare occasions, patients such as Janet Adkins feel a sense of hopelessness and choose suicide should not proscribe truth-telling. Instead, it should motivate health care professionals to provide better comfort and support systems for patients and their caregivers. Second, the lack of absolute certainty about diagnosis and prognosis is intrinsic to medicine. Once a doctor is fairly certain about a diagnosis (often evidenced by treatment choices and information shared with the family), patients should be informed. Third, although some people may argue that by the time a diagnosis is made, the patient is incompetent, there are various stages in Alzheimer's disease. In the early stages, patients may retain decisional capacity that results in a mandate for physicians to inform them so that patients can participate in decision making about medical treatment (e.g., experimental drugs) and life in general. Although physicians should be sensitive to the real fears, concerns, and even denial that patients and families may experience, family desires to withhold a diagnosis should not override the physician's primary responsibility to the patient. Compassionate disclosure can aid in ameliorating such concerns. As the ability to diagnose the disease improves clinically and new treatments emerge, doctors will have to become more comfortable with the disclosure of this troubling diagnosis.

As a patient enters the middle stages of the disease process, the capacity to participate in decision making diminishes greatly. Even so, at this stage of the disease, patients may suffer from depression and anxiety that indicate that although they may not fully understand, they still "feel" what is going on. Therefore, information about diagnosis and treatment still may have the capacity to affect a patient's life in a beneficial fashion. The physician and family are instrumental in judging whether such is the case. The extent to which a patient will understand and retain this information varies, but the effort to include the patient reinforces a fundamental respect for the patient as a person living with a disease process that robs the patient of self-determination. In the final stages of Alzheimer's, when a patient has progressed so far in the disease process that no possible meaning or purpose could be derived from any information, there is no obligation to disclose this "futile" knowledge (futile in the sense that the patient's incapacity makes it unusable). The physician's clinical judgment and the caregiver's experience indicate when information no longer provides the capacity for patient benefit.

Conclusion

Physicians have a certain latitude and discretion regarding how and when to tell patients and families a diagnosis. After the patient and family have a chance to assimilate the information, follow-up visits should be scheduled to allow for questions and concerns to be raised. Families and physicians should resist the temptation to withhold information out of fear of the disease and the effect of disclosure on the patient. Such worries may be projections that may lead to a conspiracy of silence—which, in turn, results in further isolation of the patient. The presumption for disclosure and openness serves to strengthen the physician-patient relationship and ultimately may help to reduce some of the fears associated with diseases such as Alzheimer's.

Chapter 75 _____
Ethics Committees in Hospitals

The American Hospital Association (AHA) recommends that each hospital institute an ethics committee. The action of the AHA may be an outgrowth of the study of ethics committees published by the President's Commission for Ethics in Medicine and Behavioral and Biomedical Research. Although the President's Commission stopped short of recommending that an ethics committee be established in each hospital, it clearly recommended that education, consultation, and review be available in each hospital for difficult decisions of patient care. The Joint Commission for the Accreditation of Health Care Facilities (JCAHF) also requires the availability of ethical consultation. In view of the recommendations of these three influential groups, this chapter considers the purpose and functions of ethics committees in hospitals and evaluates their usefulness.

Principles

Ethics committees in hospitals received their main impetus from the decision of the New Jersey Supreme Court in the Karen Ann Quinlan case. The court, assuming erroneously that most hospitals already had ethics committees, declared that such committees rather than the courts should be involved in decisions concerning withdrawal of life-support systems. At about the same time, the President's Commission listed six potential functions of ethical committees in hospitals:

1. Review a case to confirm the physician's diagnosis or prognosis of a patient's condition.
2. Review decisions made by physicians or surrogates about specific treatment.
3. Make decisions about suitable treatment for incompetent patients.
4. Provide general educational programs for staff on how to identify and solve ethical issues.
5. Formulate policies to be followed by staff in certain difficult cases.
6. Serve as consultant for physicians, patients, or their families in making specific ethical decisions.

Discussion

Clearly, the last three functions are educational; they could be carried out with regard to routine ethical issues as well as crisis situations. The first three functions are not educational; they could be termed jurisdictional powers because they bespeak a review power and, in some cases, a decision-making power. These jurisdictional powers are needed, the commission maintains, in ethical cases that involve the medical treatment of incompetent patients who are in danger of death. For example, an ethics committee with these powers might be called on to affirm or deny medical opinions that a patient is in a coma, make a decision about withdrawing life-support equipment, or review the decision-making process to ensure that all concerned people were consulted.

Hence, the Quinlan court and the AHA are interested in having hospitals form ethics committees with jurisdictional powers. The main concern of the court seems to be that cases involving treatment for incompetent moribund patients be settled in the hospitals rather than in the courts. One concern of the AHA seems to be that costs be controlled by removing life-support systems as soon as possible, while necessary safeguards to avoid malpractice suits are observed.

Although the concerns of the court and the AHA are legitimate, there are difficulties that accompany giving jurisdictional power to a committee within a hospital. First, it may remove medical and ethical decisions from the persons who are responsible for the decisions. In caring for dying people, whether competent or incompetent, physicians have the responsibility to make ethical decisions based on medical facts. Responsibility for discerning these medical facts cannot be given to other persons nor to a committee. The patient—or the patient's family, if the patient is incompetent—also has ethical responsibilities that should not be delegated.

Second, giving review or decision-making power to the ethics committee may dilute the ethical decision-making process rather than improve it by weakening concern for the good of the patient. Everybody's business is nobody's business. In referring ethical decisions to a committee, there is built-in potential for enervating the decision-making process by emphasizing secondary factors such as economic concerns.

Third, the introduction of a review system for treatment of patients at the time of death could lead to a wider review system of all cases, with cost-control implications. The use of high technology in diagnosing patients' conditions could be subject to these committees as well. In sum, placing jurisdictional review or decision-making powers in the hands of the ethics committee may not lead to better treatment of people who are in danger of death.

Perhaps the ethics committee would be able to fulfill its purpose through educational functions alone, however. Formal health care education in the recent past has not prepared people for competent ethical decision making, and the situation is not likely to improve in the immediate future. The solution to this perceived lack of preparation, however, is not to put ethical decision making in the hands of a few people. Instead, health care professionals should have "on-the-job" opportunities to assimilate general and specific knowledge pertinent to ethical decision making. This education can be provided through workshops, case studies, and consultation in individual cases, so that health care professionals can acquire the knowledge necessary for ethical decision making.

In addition, knowledge may be enhanced if the ethics committee outlines policies—to be approved and put into effect through the usual administrative process—for specific ethical problems. For example, several hospitals are formulating policies on withholding cardiopulmonary resuscitation. These policies do not remove the ethical responsibilities from the concerned persons: instead, they ensure more effective personal decision making because they set the limits within which such ethical decisions will be made.

Conclusion

Decisions concerning the care of people who are near death, whether those persons are old or newborn, involve many medical and ethical difficulties. There is no way to ensure that such decisions will be easy, but we can ensure that, insofar as is humanly possible, such decisions will be well-informed and responsible and made with the benefit of the patient as the foremost and determining factor. Given the history of health care and medicine and the tendency toward impersonal decision making by the committee process, all concerned parties will be better served if the responsibility for decision making rests with physicians, patients, and patients' families rather than with an ethics committee.

Chapter 76 _____

The Role of Ethics Committees

An empirical study of ethics committees in hospitals found that ethics committees are used for everything from "acting as a public relations tool for justifying unpopular decisions resulting from discontinuing unprofitable services to serving as an alternative to the courts."[1] Although most ethics committees have a more limited purview, the study revealed that many ethics committees believe they should be involved at some time in particular medical decisions concerning patient care.

On the basis of considerations of the nature of the physician-patient relationship, this chapter discusses the responsibility for ethical decision making in medicine. The discussion attempts to set forth realistic guidelines for the activities of ethics committees.

Principles

Physicians promise to help patients avoid illness, regain health, or live with infirmity as vitally as possible. The objectives of the physician-patient relationship always presuppose that the physician will offer help in accord with the patient's personal values. Thus, medicine is not an abstract science dealing only with scientific principles to particular individuals. The social and spiritual dimensions of the persons to whom scientific principles are applied, as well as their varying desires and needs, make the inclusion of values a necessity in forming a medical plan. For this reason, Leon Kass maintains that medicine, by its very nature, is a moral enterprise.[2]

In the recent past, some philosophers have maintained that in science one cannot progress logically from the "is" to the "ought," from the scientific to the ethical. Thus, they maintain, science and its applications are "value free"; the moral dimension of scientific and medical judgments is added from other disciplines. If values are intrinsic to decisions concerning medical care, however, there is no reason to assume that a transition must be made from "is" to "ought." The "ought"—the ethical dimension—is an integral part of the medical decision.

Physicians and patients (or patient proxies) have something to contribute to the medical care decision. The patient or proxy primarily expresses the desires and values of the person seeking medical help. The physician mainly makes a diagnosis and designs a medical care program in accord with the expressed wishes of the patient. The medical care decision is a cooperative product that is based on mutual trust.

What role does medical ethics have in this description of medical decision making? Medical ethics is not a new subspecialty within medicine. Physicians—not ethicists or ethics committees— are responsible for ensuring that the ethical perspective is present in medical decisions. Maintaining that physicians decide one aspect of patient care and ethicists another presents a caricature of medicine and ethics. Although ethicists can help physicians prepare for medical decision making in accord with accepted ethical norms, ethicists can never replace physicians.

What are accepted ethical norms? Obtaining informed consent for therapy is an example of an accepted ethical norm for medical care. Ethicists help physicians understand the essential elements of informed consent, but physicians ensure that informed consent is obtained.

Another accepted ethical norm of medical care states that physicians should not induce death, although they allow patients to die in certain circumstances. Helping physicians understand the circumstances that allow them to apply this important but subtle norm is the role of the ethicist. Although a body of knowledge exists that justifies calling medical ethics a distinct discipline— and thus justifies the role of medical ethicists—there is no reason to make the medical ethicist a principal participant in medical decision making. In general, the medical ethicist acts as an educator and, in specific cases, as a consultant, which is simply a more personal form of education.

If we are to preserve the integrity of the physician-patient relationship, the ethics committee should be envisioned as a group of persons fulfilling the rule of the medical ethicist. Thus, the committee should offer to health care professionals and their patients only education and consultation.

Discussion

With this slightly more limited function assigned to medical ethics and ethics committees, several observations are in order.

- Ethics committees should devote intense activity to self-education. If the committee is to sponsor education and consultation according to accepted ethical principles, its members must be knowledgeable about the principles in question. Common sense does not suffice for sound ethical decisions. The President's Commission for the Study of Ethical Problems in Medicine and Biomedical and Behavioral Research has developed some principles for our pluralistic society.[3] The Catholic Church, in accord with its notion of the nature of the human person, has also developed ethical norms for medical care. Depending on the character of the health care facility, the ethics committee should school itself in one or both of these sets of principles.

- The ethics committee need not include people from "all walks of life." When hospitals draw up criteria for ethics committees, they tend to require persons who are "nonscientific," persons who "represent the community," or persons who are "consumers of health care." Clearly, when membership of "outsiders" on ethics committees is recommended, there is a possibility that ethical decisions in medicine will be based on public opinion rather than on accepted ethical principles and the knowledge of medical practice. People from all walks of life may serve effectively on ethics committees in health care facilities if they are knowledgeable about ethics, but they do not qualify as ethical experts simply because they are outside the profession of health care. Persons qualify for ethics committees through their ability to analyze issues from well-reasoned ethical perspectives.

- The main purpose of ethics committees is to sponsor education programs for all persons associated with the health care facility. The formulation of policy with regard to ethical issues, such as policies for do-not-resuscitate (DNR) orders or transplantation of organs, simply represents more specific educational programs. If consultation on an ethical issue is requested by a physician or a patient (or proxy), the purpose should be to help the physician and patient sort out their thinking. The ethics committee does not replace the physician or the patient. The concept that the ethics committee becomes some sort of jury before whom evidence is presented is a travesty of ethical decision making.

Conclusion

The foregoing vision of .ethics committees does not call for a deemphasis of these committees. True, if the relationship between the physician and the patient is to be respected, ethics committees will have a more limited responsibility than some people would desire. The need for education in medical ethics should not be underemphasized, however. Physicians and other health care professionals do not know intuitively the principles of medical ethics. Thus, they require the input and expertise of the ethics committee in their ethical decision making.

Notes

1. Alister Browne, "Ethics Committees for What?" *Canadian Medical Association Journal,*136 (June 1987) 1149–57.
2. Leon Kass, *Toward a More Natural Science: Biology and Human Affairs* (New York-Free Press, 1988), 65.
3. *Deciding to Forgo Life-Sustaining Treatment*-U.S. Government Printing Office, 1983-150–56; 160–65.

Chapter 77 _____

"There but for the Grace of God": Disclosing Imperfect Care

A 1989 article in the *Journal of the American Medical Association* summarized the attitudes of a group of practicing physicians toward truth-telling. One scenario to which the doctors responded involved a situation in which the physician mistakenly administered ten times the normal dose of medication, which directly resulted in the patient's death. Only 55 percent of the physicians said they would tell the family the full truth that a mistake had been made.[1] The response to this scenario raises important ethical questions. What obligation do health care professionals have to reveal to patients or their families when they have caused harm? How serious does the harm have to be?

Principles

Very early in life, children are encouraged to "own up to mistakes" and to tell the truth, especially when damage to another's property or person is involved. Treatment programs such as Alcoholics Anonymous encourage participants to assume accountability for their actions, to ask forgiveness from people they have harmed. We expect people to leave a note if they have damaged our car in a parking lot. Two principles ground this presumption for disclosure: justice and respect for persons. The principle of justice implies that compensation is owed to people who have been unjustly harmed. Respect for persons suggests that we should be honest in our interactions with each other. A lack of truth-telling leads to distrust and deprives people of information to which they are rightly entitled. Even though we are not always obliged to reveal all of the truth we know, when people are entitled to information, concealing the truth (like a direct lie) constitutes unethical deception.

Investigating the issue of disclosure of harm requires that one define the magnitude of harm as well as the health care professional's role in causing the harm. With regard to the magnitude of harm, intuitively one would argue that actions that result in death, disability, disfigurement, serious pain, loss of wages, or additional hospitalization would be the subject of disclosure. On the other hand, if a nurse mistakenly administers 10 mg of valium instead of 5 mg, the harm seems insufficient to demand disclosure. Health care professionals must make a prudential decision for cases that fall between these endpoints. With regard to the causative role in the harm, when it is outside of the general purview of what is considered professional culpability, there is little hesitancy to reveal to patients the genesis of harm. For example, a patient with no previous history of drug allergy may react to a medication and suffer anaphylactic shock; harm may result from a known risk of a procedure that the patient knowingly undertook; or a physician may choose a treatment that falls under acceptable standards of care but in hindsight turns out to be inferior to another treatment.

The controversy over disclosure usually arises in cases in which harm results from negligent care by the health care professional. Negligent care does not imply a lack of perfect care; it involves failure to exercise due care demanded by professional standards or engagement in unethical behavior that results in direct harm to the patient. Examples would include blatant misinterpretation of an x ray, ekg, or slide; removal of the wrong organ; incorrect administration of a drug; or observation of incompetent care provided by a colleague. These types of mistake inhibit truth-telling because they require admittance of personal error or error by a colleague.

From a legal perspective, no statutes demand that health care professionals disclose negligent behavior to patients or their families. Yet there are legal consequences of failure to disclose negligent behavior to patients or families. The statute of limitations for a malpractice suit may be extended, and the jury likely will reward additional punitive damages for failure to disclose. Regardless of whether there is a positive legal duty to disclose, is there an ethical one based on the principles of respect for persons and justice?

Discussion

Health care professionals have cited several competing ethical interests to justify their failure to disclose information when they are at fault. First, they question whether such disclosure will do any good once the damage is done. Second, the revelation of mistakes to patients and families will result in a loss of confidence in the practitioner's ability, thereby creating a relationship of distrust. Third, such disclosure will increase the probability of career-threatening and expensive lawsuits. Fourth, an ethical duty to disclose would foster a climate of suspicion and distrust among fellow caregivers, which could lead to false and vengeful reporting. Moreover, health care professionals see reporting as distasteful because of the realization that "there but for the grace of God go I." Finally, health care professionals believe that internal policing will discover and discipline individuals responsible for substandard care.

At first glance, these interests seem to be compelling. Yet these concerns reflect a myopic vision that does not seem to focus primarily on the well-being and perspective of the patient. When patients have been harmed by truly negligent actions, they do have a right and an expectation to know the truth and be compensated accordingly. Many patients do not have disability insurance, whereas health care professionals do carry malpractice insurance precisely because at times they may not render "due care" and consequently may cause patient harm.

Admittedly, through disclosure patients may lose a certain confidence in their health care workers. Perhaps, however, it is time to shatter some of the unrealistic patient expectations of health care professionals. Sadly, this process may be difficult because the demand for "perfection" will continue to grow in a business-oriented, consumer/provider health system that promotes lawsuits when the "customer" is not satisfied.

Within and outside health care, people must realize that health care professionals make mistakes. Moreover, greater damage occurs to the physician-patient relationship when patients or families inadvertently discover that information has been concealed. Finally, because patients lack medical education, it is unreasonable to presume that they would know that an act of negligence has occurred. This power and knowledge differential engenders a positive obligation to disclose.

Interestingly, health care professionals readily reveal a mistake that is self evident, such as operating on the wrong knee. Likewise, health care professionals are more forthcoming if the patient or family has a medical background that would assist them in realizing that a negligent action has occurred. Thus, it seems disingenuous to withhold information in other cases simply because the patient or family lacks the wherewithal to realize the mistake.

Of course, to avoid inappropriate disclosure, when possible, health care professionals who feel they may have made a negligent error should consult appropriate superiors, colleagues, and perhaps legal counsel to verify that their actions truly did result in the harm. Disclosure need not be an admittance of legal fault but merely a revelation of truth grounded in a fundamental respect for the patient.

An extremely sensitive situation arises when a third party witnesses or becomes aware of negligent behavior by a colleague or referring health care professional. The problem is compounded by the fact that often the negligent health care professional may be unaware of his or her negligence. Reporting a colleague, even if it involves revealing the truth, subjects the reporter to potential hostility, accusations of disloyalty, and retaliation for "squealing." The internal inertia to critique has frequently enervated self-policing mechanisms in health care.

Much is at stake when one is reporting what is perceived to be negligent or unethical behavior. Of primary importance is the welfare and safety of patients who have been harmed or may be harmed in the future. Professional reputations also must be considered, however. Behavior that may appear to be negligent may in fact reflect legitimate differences of opinion about care.

Ideally, one would try to speak with the offending professional and have him or her initiate an evaluation of the problematic actions. This procedure presumes (albeit a faulty presumption at times) that health care professionals would be open to potential critique and correction from our colleagues. Failing that, professionals would have an ethical and at times legal duty to bring the mistake to the attention of a superior, quality assurance personnel, and, when applicable, the risk manager and state boards for evaluation of the behavior for the sake of patient care.

Witnesses to apparently negligent actions should avoid directly informing the patient or families. Mechanisms should be established to protect third parties from retaliation when they report negligence. Nevertheless, in institutional or private practice, internal disciplinary action to censure inappropriate care must include disclosure to the patient or family when significant harm has occurred and a direct line of causality has been established.

Conclusion

Disclosure is a complex subject. Health care professionals hold different positions about disclosure. Many values are at stake—including patient well-being, professional reputation, and collegial trust. Many health care professionals express a willingness to be forthright with patients about mistakes but feel inhibited by fears of malpractice claims and career disruption. This inhibition does not negate the ethical duty to disclose, but it suggests alternatives to current practices—including the establishment of a system similar to worker's compensation that would compensate patients appropriately, improve the quality of care for patients, and strengthen the process of internal review. At the very least, review and reform of malpractice law with regard to punitive damages may eradicate some of the inhibition to truthful disclosure of mistakes.

Ultimately, health care professionals, like all of us, must face up to the reality of our imperfection. As one physician lamented, "The potential consequences of our medical mistakes are so overwhelming that it is almost impossible for practicing physicians to deal with their errors in a psychologically healthy way."[2] The time has come to address the impossible.

Notes

1. D. Novack et al., "Physicians' Attitudes Toward Using Deception to Resolve Difficult Ethical Problems," *Journal of the American Medical Association* 261 (1989): 2982.
2. D. Hilfiker, "Facing Our Mistakes," *NEJM* 310 (1984): 3448–51.

Chapter 78 _____

Treatment of Rape Victims

Two events bring the question of ethical treatment of rape victims into consideration. The first event is the development of a true "morning after pill": RU486, an extremely effective method of terminating pregnancy within the first nine weeks of gestation. Second, an appellate court in California ruled that Catholic hospitals have the responsibility "to provide information concerning, and access to, estrogen prophylaxis for rape victims.[1]" Because the court case involved Catholic hospitals, this chapter considers the proper treatment of rape victims from the perspective of Catholic teaching.

Principles

A victim of rape should be given the most sensitive and charitable care possible. Rape victims often complain—justifiably—that they are treated by the police and medical personnel alike as though they were responsible for provoking the attack, thus compounding the grave injustice the woman has suffered. Hospital procedures for the treatment of rape victims should be designed to accomplish four goals:

- Offer psychological support and counseling that the woman needs to work through the trauma of the attack and its aftermath.
- Provide medical care for injuries or abrasions that might have occurred.
- Gather evidence to be used to help in apprehending and prosecuting the rapist.
- Provide treatment to prevent possible sexually transmitted disease and pregnancy.

This last point—preventing pregnancy—raises special ethical problems. Avoiding pregnancy is a very serious concern for a rape victim, and she deserves all the help that medical professionals can give—provided that the help is ethical. In many cases, it will be possible to determine that conception is not feasible—for example, if the woman is taking contraceptive drugs or if an examination of cervical mucus shows that she is not in a fertile phase. If pregnancy is a possibility, however, the victim—who is in no way responsible for the possible pregnancy—has the right to avoid conception. A woman who has consented to intercourse takes responsibility as a free person to use the sexual act in keeping with its intrinsic significance of love and procreation. A rape victim has no such responsibility because she has not consented to the sexual act. However, according to Catholic teaching, once a woman has conceived, she cannot take any direct action to abort or to destroy a fertilized ovum or request others to do so.[2] Because a fertilized ovum is a human being, albeit in an incipient stage, it deserves the respect owed to human life. Ethical problems arise, then, when hospitals use methods to prevent conception that may have the effect of preventing conception but that also may cause the destruction of a fertilized ovum if conception has already occurred.

Discussion

In the United States, most hospital rape protocols recommend the administration of antifertility drugs such as Ovral in large dosage (100 mg) within seventy-two hours of the rape; a second dose is taken twelve hours later. The rape protocols specify that Ovral or other estrogenic hormones should not be administered until a test is given to determine if the woman is pregnant. If the pregnancy test is positive, the pregnancy occurred before the rape, and treatment with Ovral may injure the embryo.

May rape protocols that call for the administration of Ovral be utilized in a Catholic hospital? Ovral and similar estrogenic compounds have two effects: They inhibit ovulation, but they also impede implantation of the embryo if fertilization has already occurred. Hence, if Ovral is given with the intention of inhibiting ovulation and preventing conception, its use is acceptable—provided it is given at a time in the woman's cycle when it could prevent ovulation or impede the motility of the sperm and thus prevent fertilization. Hence, any antifertility medication must be given within seventy-two hours of the rape. Otherwise, the effect of the medication would be useless in preventing conception because the sperm would be inactive or dead. If the antiovulatory medication is given at a time in the menstrual cycle when its only effect would be to prevent implantation of the fertilized ovum, its use would not be acceptable. The principle of double effect justifies the use of Ovral or similar medications if the intention is to avoid conception and the medication is given at a time in the woman's cycle when ovulation has not occurred.

What if there is doubt about whether the woman has ovulated (a situation that would be true of many women who present themselves for treatment after rape)? A Catholic ethics committee in Great Britain asked this question and responded—rightly it seems—that if there is doubt about whether ovulation has occurred within the present menstrual cycle, antifertility drugs may be used with the intention of preventing ovulation because the probability that fertilization has occurred is minimal. The doubt in question concerns the fact of ovulation, not the fact of conception.

Ovral and other estrogenic hormones that inhibit ovulation are entirely different from RU486, the true "morning after pill." When used after intercourse, RU486 has *only* an abortifacient effect. RU486 produces its effect by blocking the normal action of the hormone progesterone, thus preventing implantation of the fertilized ovum. Hence, in care for rape victims, RU486 is not an alternative for Catholic hospitals. At present, RU486 is sold commercially only in France and China; how long it will remain unavailable in other countries is unclear. Much confusion has been generated by courts, lawyers, and health care professionals who use the term "morning after pill" to refer to medications that are utilized with the intention of preventing conception. A firm distinction should be made between antiovulatory medications, such as Ovral, and RU486.

Conclusion

What is the import of the decision of the California appeals court insofar as Catholic hospitals are concerned? First, the California court declared that the hospital has a responsibility to provide "information concerning, and access to, estrogen pregnancy prophylaxis" for rape victims. It allowed the hospital to fulfill this responsibility "by instructing the patient concerning the options for pregnancy prevention and by transferring the patient to another medical facility or another physician." Yet Catholic hospitals appear to be justified in offering direct service to rape victims. Hence, every Catholic hospital should have an explicit policy that delineates the circumstances in which antifertility medications may be used to help rape victims avoid conception.[3] Second, the concept of abortion put forward by the California appeals court is not acceptable from the perspective of Catholic teaching. The court considers efforts to prevent implantation of a fertilized ovum to be "birth control," whereas Catholic teaching considers this effort to be abortion. A better effort to present to the court the scientific evidence maintaining that a fertilized ovum is a human being, even before implantation, seems to be in order.

Notes

1. Second Appellate District of California: *Brownfield v. Daniel Freeman Marine Hospital,* March 2, 1989.
2. National Conference of Catholic Bishops, (NCCB), *Ethical and Religious Directives,* vol. 36 (Washington D.C., 1995).
3. Committee on Bioethical issues for the Bishops of Great Britain & Ireland, "Use of the Morning After Pill in Rape Cases," *Origins* (March 13, 1986): 633.633–38.

Chapter 79 _____

Separating the Lakeberg Twins: Ethical Issues

Amy and Angela Lakeberg were born at Loyola University Medical Center in Maywood, Illinois, a suburb of Chicago. Before their birth, their parents learned that the twins were joined at the chest. Upon delivery, they learned that the twins shared a heart and liver. In the opinion of the neonatal physicians at Loyola, both would soon die if they were not separated. Moreover, even if they were separated, the chance of keeping the surviving twin alive was judged to be less than 1 percent. The parents, after being informed by the Loyola physicians of the situation, asked to have the twins separated, in the hope that one would survive. Accordingly, a surgical team from Children's Hospital in Philadelphia—which had operated on several other sets of conjoined twins in recent years, agreed to accept the case. Surgery was performed in Philadelphia in August 1993. As a result of the effort to position a functioning heart in the body of one of the twins, Amy died immediately, and Angela died shortly thereafter.

After delivery, as well as before and after the surgery to separate the twins, a discussion was carried on in the media concerning the ethical issues arising from the Lakeberg case. In this chapter our interest is directed toward these issues.

Effective Surgery?

The first ethical issue in the Lakeberg case is whether to perform surgery. Moreover, we have to evaluate the surgery as therapy and as a research project. Insofar as therapy is concerned, surgery should be performed if it is judged likely to be effective and does not impose a grave burden. Surgery is effective if it will enable the patient—in this case the twins—to pursue the purpose of life. That is, would the surgery enable the twins to think, love, relate to others, and pursue the goods of life that are associated with human fulfillment? Clearly, although surgery alone will not help a person strive for the purpose of life, it can establish a physiological basis for this endeavor.

In answering the question concerning the effectiveness of the surgery, we are faced immediately with the realization that one of the twins must die as a result of the surgery. Thus, the surgery would not be effective insofar as the nonsurviving twin was concerned. Because doctors foresaw that Amy would die, some people condemned the surgery because they said it would involve killing Amy to save Angela. On the other hand, this situation seems to be a classic case of the principle of double effect. The object of the moral action is to save Angela through surgery; in the course of performing this action, because of the position of the shared organs an unwanted effect necessarily occurs—namely, the death of Amy. From the point of view of Amy's death, then, it does not seem that the surgery involves a direct killing.

Is the surgery effective from the point of view of Angela? This question is difficult to answer because her prognosis is so uncertain. The neonatologists at Loyola and the surgeons in Philadelphia did not offer more hope of success than a 1 percent chance. Thus, there was a 99 percent chance of failure. Moreover, we have no idea of what the possibility of "success" implied. Would the surgery be considered successful simply if Angela survived after the surgery for a few weeks or months? Would the surgery be successful if Angela were respirator-dependent for years to come and would need to remain in an institution? How would neurological deficit be reckoned insofar as success is concerned? Although the meaning of "success" is difficult to determine insofar as the surgery is concerned—given the uncertainty of Angela's survival for any length of time and the debilitated condition that would probably ensue after surgery, saying that the surgery had a 1 percent chance of success seems a bit optimistic.

Excessive Burden?

Even if some people would judge the surgery to be potentially effective for Angela, it must also be evaluated insofar as the burden it imposes is concerned. The burden of any medical therapy must be considered from the point of view of the patient, as well as from the point of view of the family and society. When we consider the burden from the point of view of Angela, we consider not only the burden of the surgery but also the burden that will be imposed on her in the future as a result of the surgery. With regard to the surgery itself, it doesn't seem to have imposed an excessive burden. Did the surgery impose an excessive burden insofar as Angela's future life is concerned? This question is difficult to decide because of the vagueness of the prognosis and the uncertainty of her function and survival. Even if the surgery were to allow Angela to survive, would that survival be beneficial or burdensome? At the time of the surgery, no one could say. Yet how many ventures would a prudent person pursue if the hope for success were less than 1 percent?

Can the burden be deemed excessive insofar as the parents are concerned? Reitha and Ken Lakeberg seemed willing to assume the burden associated with caring for Angela. Hence, it would be difficult to assert excessive burden insofar as the parents are concerned. Insofar as society is concerned, the main objection to the surgery concerned the money that would be spent on the care of the twins in tertiary care facilities in Maywood and Philadelphia. Many observers asked, "Couldn't that money be put to better use—for example, by devoting it to prenatal care?"

The fact is, if the money were not devoted to the care of the twins it would not be devoted to prenatal care. Our society has a very convoluted method of funding health care for catastrophic cases like the Lakeberg's. Funding of health care results from an amalgam of public, private, and charitable sources that are unpredictable but often provide the necessary funds. Although this situation does not seem to be the optimal method of funding health care, it is the method that exists in our society at present. Thus, the physicians and hospital administrators who cared for the Lakeberg twins can not be faulted for a misuse of resources once they decided to perform the surgery. The surgeon in Philadelphia seems to be justified in saying, "If someone is going to ration health care because of money, it is not going to be us." In the future, society may wish to address the economic implications of catastrophic treatment in a more reasonable manner, but at present, surgeons do not have the responsibility of allocating funds for catastrophic cases.

Research

If the surgery were deemed ineffective or excessively burdensome as a medical procedure, could it be justified as a research project? Research, in the strict sense of the term, does not aim at healing or curing but at acquiring new knowledge for the good of humanity. Of course, research is often combined with therapy; in such cases, the overall project does have a healing or curing purpose. In the strict sense, however, research seeks to gain knowledge that will benefit people in the future. Although one can accept serious risk of harm for oneself and thus volunteer for research projects in the strict sense of the term, the ethical validity of proxy consent does not allow one person to put another person at risk of serious harm unless there is hope of therapeutic benefit. When the ethical issues of the Lakeberg case were discussed, some people expressed the view that the surgery was justified because it might provide knowledge for the future. The risk to the twins, especially to Amy, was too great, however, to justify the surgery under the aegis of research. The history of research on humans, from Auschwitz to Tuskeegee, is replete with examples of subjects and researchers who are dehumanized as a result of research without informed consent.

Decision Makers

Finally, who has the ethical right and responsibility to make decisions concerning the medical care of the Lakeberg twins? The first response to this question might be the parents because the children were not able to offer consent for themselves. This response is a bit shortsighted, however, because when making any type of reasonable decision parents will require medical information from the physicians involved in the case. Thus, informed consent, especially in the case of infants, is a collaborative decision. The physicians must make a decision about whether the surgery would seem to be effective and offer this information to the parents.

Insofar as ethical medicine is concerned, the physicians have the right and often the obligation to declare that a particular therapy is futile and that they do not offer that particular therapy as an option. Unfortunately, physicians seldom make a declaration that a particular therapy is futile if the parents or proxies of incapacitated patients vehemently request such therapy. The mentality of the physicians in the Lakeberg case was evidenced by a surgeon in Philadelphia who stated that the main reason for performing the surgery was the Lakeberg's wishes: "We take the position that the parents have the right to choose for their children." This claim is true in most cases—but not if the surgery is likely to be ineffective (in the opinion of the surgeons). A more collaborative decision might have yielded a different decision in the Lakeberg case.

Conclusion

The most disconcerting aspect of the Lakeberg case is the realization that ethical decisions often must be made with incomplete and insufficient information. Under those circumstances, there is no moral mandate to pursue the course of action that might prolong life, especially if there is only insignificant hope of success. As Daniel Callahan remarked, "The yoking of sanctity of life and the technological imperative has led to the common conclusion that, when in doubt, we should treat." The ethical reality, however, is that actions need not be performed if the hope of success is very remote. Hence, there is no ethical mandate to do whatever is possible; instead, there is a mandate to do what is reasonable. With this perspective in mind—not because millions of dollars were expended—the decisions made to separate the Lakeberg twins may be called into question.

Chapter 80

The McCaughey Septuplets: All's Well that Ends Well?

A few years have passed since Bobbi McCaughey successfully gave birth to septuplets. Though the infants were born at only thirty weeks gestation, all of the babies weighed more than 1,000 grams and had relatively uncomplicated stays in the hospital. The McCaugheys, now out of the national limelight, must go about the task of raising the septuplets and their other daughter with the help of friends and the community in Carlisle, Iowa. Although random chance seemingly operated in this couple's favor, this world-famous birthing event and the circumstances that led up to it require ethical evaluation. Two specific areas of analysis involve how we create or transmit human life and the respect for persons brought into existence by techniques of assisted reproduction.

Principles

The McCaughey case caused people to question some of their underlying assumptions about the responsible use of reproductive technologies. The inviolable nature of reproductive liberty and the "right" to have a child have unquestionably governed the contemporary use of reproductive technologies by couples and individuals. In the wake of a sixty-three-year old woman giving birth; designer embryos for sale; a fraternal twin born eight years after his sibling; the specter of human cloning looming on the horizon; and this septuplet case, people have begun to question the norms that have supported our libertine approach to reproduction.

Undue emphasis on freedom and rights risks devaluing and violating the nature of human procreation. This emphasis also potentially threatens to undermine our respect for the human beings brought into existence because they are no longer viewed as the primary focus of ethical concern. An appropriate use of reproductive technologies must entail a respect for the intrinsic nature of the procreative process in the context of conjugal intercourse. Simply because a technology or process can transmit or create life does not create an ethical warrant for its use. The end does not justify all possible means to that end.

Technological interventions or treatments that enhance rather than distort or replace our nature best promote human flourishing and would be deemed ethically acceptable. Moreover, this respect for and willingness to work with our nature and its internal *telos* must be accompanied by a respect for the fruits of that nature—the children called into existence. Arguments that speak of a "right" to a child already betray a lack of respect for the child, who is viewed as an object of ownership. People do not have a right to a child. Couples plan their families responsibly and have children as an expression of love in light of their particular circumstances and abilities.

Discussion

In the McCaughey case and others like it, couples confront the choice of using fertility drugs to overcome reproductive difficulties. The use of fertility drugs does not include the additional difficulties traditionally associated with techniques such as IVF, GIFT, and ICSI in terms of the nature of the transmission of human life. That is, drugs used to promote fertility clearly enhance rather than replace or distort the natural process of procreation. Because of the risk for multifetal pregnancy attached to the use of fertility drugs, however, one must ethically discern whether such treatment shows appropriate respect for the life that is called into being.

Less powerful drugs such as Clomed can result in multiple gestations in 6–8 percent of cases (almost exclusively cases of twinning). More powerful drugs such as Pergonal or Metrodin (the drug used by the McCaugheys) produce multiple gestations at rates of about 25 percent; one-third of the multiple gestations produce triplets or higher-order pregnancies. The risk of multiple fertilization can be decreased by carefully monitoring follicular maturation. If it appears that multiple eggs will be released by the developing follicles, the chemical trigger to release the eggs can be withheld, and the couple then waits for a more opportune cycle to attempt to become pregnant. However, given the cost of treatment and monitoring—$2,000–$3,000 per cycle—couples often risk a possible multifetal pregnancy.

What considerations should enter into a couple's decision to try to become pregnant in such circumstances? Is this situation even an ethical concern? As one physician in the McCaughey case asked, "Should we as a society dictate to individuals the size of their families or their choices of reproductive care?" Do couples have a right to gamble? In response, if respect for the children brought into existence represents the fundamental norm of discernment, the decision does have societal as well as individual ethical implications when a multifetal pregnancy is a significant possibility.

Multifetal pregnancies—particularly those that involve more than triplets—can cause health risks for the mother, such as an increased risk for hypertension, gestational diabetes, and anemia, as well as side effects from tocolytic agents that often are used to stop premature contractions. For the children, the initial risks are morbidity and mortality associated with the extreme prematurity that accompanies a higher-order multifetal pregnancy. Although advances in neonatal care have substantially increased the odds of survival, very high order multifetal pregnancies still can result in the death of several of the children and severe impairment for the survivors. In essence, the McCaugheys were incredibly fortuitous to have had such a good outcome.

Besides those immediate risks and their long-term physical sequelae, higher-order multifetal pregnancies generally result in great physical, emotional, and financial stress on families, including an increased risk for divorce. As a mother of triplets commented, "I think the woman in Iowa is totally nuts. And if she's not nuts now, she will be."

Finally, there is a social cost. The hospital bill for the McCaugheys will no doubt approach or even exceed $1 million. Had there been greater morbidity or impairment, the initial and long-terms costs would have been even higher. One could argue that some pregnancies by chance result in high costs, and society does not balk at financing such care. When powerful fertility drugs are employed, however, the parents forseeably risk the complications. Is it fair for society to have to pay for expensive outcomes resulting from voluntary interventions by the couple?

Given the potential for harm to all parties involved and the substantial risk of a bad outcome, there is legitimate ethical concern about attempting pregnancy when it may involve a higher-order multiple gestation. Given the fact that there are accurate methods to determine if too many eggs are ripening, couples should exercise caution in such cases, despite the potential financial cost associated with having to delay until a more opportune reproductive cycle emerges.

Selective Abortion

If a high-order multifetal pregnancy does occur, what responsibility does the couple have toward the developing children? Because prematurity increases dramatically with each additional child, higher-order pregnancies have increased morbidity and, beyond quintuplets, much higher mortality. For that medical reason and other social reasons, physicians offer couples the option of reducing the number of fetuses through selective abortion—often eliminating all but two of the fetuses. Thus, couples confront the tragically ironic and ethically challenging conundrum of killing the very offspring they desperately desired in order to guarantee the survival of some.

The McCaugheys chose not to utilize selective abortion because of religious reasons. Is there also an ethical basis for that stance? The following analysis assumes that direct abortion is a moral evil. Obviously, that assumption is controversial in our society, but for those who see abortion as a legitimate practice, the issue of selective abortion is a moot point. The ethical complexity of this case arises for people who are generally opposed to abortion but could envision this case as exceptional.

Intuitively, sacrificing some of the fetuses rather than losing them all makes sense from a utilitarian standpoint. Proper ethical analysis of the issue, however, requires that a distinction be made between physical evil and moral evil. Losing seven children as opposed to five is a greater physical evil. By and large, we have an ethical duty to minimize physical evil when possible. Nevertheless, the minimization of physical evil cannot result directly from the performance of a moral evil. Thus, although the conclusion seems counterintuitive, it is ethically better to allow the natural death of seven children than to preserve two children by aborting five. Although the remote end to save the lives of the siblings is noble, the proximate intention is to kill the developing children.

Conclusion

Couples who are desperate to have children will go to great lengths and assume many risks to achieve a pregnancy. Fertility drugs have been a blessing for many couples because they allow them to have children. Yet even seemingly innocuous approaches to overcoming of infertility—such as fertility drugs—are fraught with ethical dilemmas. The McCaughey septuplet case has served as a catalyst to analyze several ethical issues. Through good luck and sound medical care, the McCaughey case has turned out well. Many experts warned other couples that this case was unusual—comparing the odds of success with the odds of winning the lottery. Therefore, couples who are at risk for high-order multifetal pregnancies because of the use of powerful fertility drugs must take into account not only their own desires for a child but the potential effects on the children, the family, and society as a whole.

Chapter 81

Early Delivery of Anencephalic Infants: Ethical Opinions

A group of obstetricians, neonatal care nurses, social workers, and ethicists representing health care facilities with neonatal care units, recently gathered to discuss early delivery of anencephalic infants. Over a period of six months, the group discussed the issue from medical, nursing, familial, and ethical perspectives. This chapter considers the issue from an ethical perspective grounded in the Catholic tradition.

Principles

This discussion presumes that a certain diagnosis of anencephaly has been made by competent specialists. This diagnosis implies that the infant in question has a debilitated cerebral cortex that will not develop sufficiently for the infant to perform human acts.

Human acts (*actus humanus,* i.e., acts of intellect and will) are distinguished from acts of man (*actus hominis,* i.e., acts of the autonomic nervous system), such as breathing or the heartbeat (cf. *Summa Theol.* I–II, q. 1, a. 1). Given that the goal of human life is to know and love God and neighbor, the distinction between human acts and acts of man is important. There is no moral obligation to prolong the life of a person who will never again be able to perform human acts because this person cannot strive to pursue the purpose of life. On the other hand, such a person may not be directly killed because doing so would be murder.

In the Catholic tradition, an anencephalic infant is a human being because it has a life principle that informs the body of the infant, even though organs of the body are not able to provide the matter for the form of the person to function properly. There is a substantial union between body and spirit (soul), even if the body cannot be the substratum for certain spiritual activities of the soul, such as knowing and loving.

In moral activity, it is important to distinguish between the goal of the action (moral object, or *finis operis*) and the goal of the agent (*finis operantis*). The goal of the action is the "what" of the human action; it specifies the morality of the human act. The goal of the agent is the "why" of the agent (cf. *Summa Theol.* I–II, q. 18, a. 6). Although both are important in judging whether human acts are good or bad, a good *finis operantis* does not excuse a bad *finis operis*.

When we seek to discern the morality of human acts, we often use the term "intention." It is important to distinguish between the proximate and remote intention (*Summa Theol.* I–II, q. 1, a. 3). The proximate intention is associated with the *finis operis;* the remote intention is associated with the *finis operantis.* G.E.M. Anscombe describes the moral object as the "intention in the action you are actually performing, whatever ulterior intentions you may have."[1] This approach seems to be an accurate manner of studying our moral actions.

In discussing the morality of early delivery of anencephalic infants, we are not concerned with the *finis operantis.* Clearly, the remote intention of parents or medical professionals who seek to deliver an anencephalic infant before the time of natural birth is good. They wish to eliminate anxiety and emotional suffering on the part of the parents of the baby. Thus, the question concerns the proximate intention inherent in the act of early delivery: the *finis operis,* or moral object. Does this act constitute a direct abortion, or is there some way to explain it as an indirect abortion?

The difference between a direct and an indirect abortion is significant. A direct abortion occurs when the *finis operis* is the death of the fetus (infant). Although other goods (*finis operantis*) may be accomplished by this action, the moral object of this act is the death of the infant. An indirect abortion occurs when the goal of the act (*finis operis*) is therapeutic benefit to the pregnant woman and the death of the fetus is a necessary but undesired effect of the therapeutic procedure. The distinction between a direct and an indirect abortion is an application of the principle of double effect.

Ethical Opinions Concerning Early Delivery of Anencephalic Infants

Thomas Boles asserts that the anencephalic infant is not a person because it will never possess cognitive-affective function.[2] Thus, it may be removed from the womb as soon as a diagnosis of anencephaly has been determined. This opinion seems to be contrary to the teaching of the Catholic Church in the document *Donum Vitae.*[3]

James Drane states that the anencephalic infant is a human person but may be delivered as soon as it is viable—about twenty-five weeks—because it will not develop any further as a human person.[4] In response to this opinion, abortion is measured not in light of viability but in light of the object of the act. Delivering an anencephalic infant after twenty-five weeks will still result in its death because it will not survive on its own and it will not receive special help (e.g. an incubator) to help its survive. Hence, the *finis operis* of the delivery (the inherent proximate intention of the act) even after viability seems to be killing an innocent human being. Moreover, early delivery of a viable infant is justified only if the infant can no longer live in the womb.[5]

Several potential pathologies may accompany a full-term delivery of anencephalic infants.[6] Could the anencephalic infant be delivered early to avoid these pathologies? This opinion would seek to invoke the principle of double effect.[7] To use the principle of double effect legitimately, however, early delivery must be an *indirect* effect of a physical procedure employed to avoid potential pathologies. The direct killing of the infant may not be the means to avoid pathologies. Hence, the application of the principle of double effect does not seem to justify the early delivery of anencephalic infants. (This conclusion is a reversal of the opinion of O'Rourke and De Blois cited above.)

Another opinion is expressed as follows: The natural purpose of pregnancy is to allow the fetus to develop into a person who will be able to perform human acts and pursue the purpose of life. At the time of the diagnosis of anencephaly, it is clear that the purpose of the pregnancy will not be fulfilled. Thus, prolonging the pregnancy is useless. Hence, the pregnancy may be terminated by removing the fetus and the surrounding matter from the womb of the mother. The problem with this opinion is that terminating a "useless pregnancy" involves a direct killing of a human person, even though the person is severely debilitated. Clearly, one need not prolong the life of an anencephalic infant because he or she will benefit from prolonged life. Is one allowed to perform an act in which either the *finis operis* or *finis operantis* is to kill a human person? If this option were licit, any dying person could be smothered or put to death directly.

To avoid spiritual or emotional pain to the mother or father, Drane maintains that when a diagnosis is made that the fetus will be anencephalic, the pregnancy may be terminated. This conclusion is an inaccurate application of the principle of totality. Trying to circumvent emotional harm—the *finis operantis* of the termination of the pregnancy—does not allow the direct killing of the infant.

Daniels[8] maintains that the womb of the pregnant woman may be considered a form of life support, similar to any medical device. Just as life-prolonging therapy such as a respirator may be removed to allow a person to die of an underlying pathology that cannot be circumvented, the anencephalic infant may be removed from its life support, the womb. Considering the womb as a life-support device seems to be a gross equivocation, however. Natural organs may not be excised or rendered inoperative unless they are diseased or in some way threaten the health or life of a patient. Anencephaly does not threaten the life of the infant nor of the mother.

Because intervention in the pregnancy of an anencephalic infant seems to result in direct killing of an innocent human being, the only suitable ethical procedure seems to be to allow the pregnancy to go to full term, baptize the infant, and allow the parents to hold it before it dies.[9]

In 1996 the Committee on Doctrine of the National Association of Catholic Bishops issued a directive that stated, "The fact that the life of a child suffering from anencephaly will probably be brief cannot excuse directly causing death before viability or gravely endangering the child's life after viability as a result of the complications of prematurity."[10]

Notes

1. "You Can Have Sex without Children: Christianity and the New Order." *Collected Philosophical Papers* (Oxford, U.K.: Basil Blackwell, 1981), 86.

2. Thomas Boles, "The Licitness (according to Roman Catholic premises) of Inducing the Non-viable Anencephalic Infant: Reflection on Professor Drane's Policy Proposals," *HEC's Forum* 4 (February1992) 121–33.

3. Congregation for the Doctrine of the Faith (CDF), *Donum Vitae*, "On Respect for Human Life," *Origins* 16 (March 19, 1987):40.

4. James Drane, "Anencephaly and the Interruption of Pregnancy: Policy Proposals for HCES," *HEC Forum* 4 (February 1992): 103–19.

5. Ethical and Religious Directives, Directive 49 Washington, D.C.: United States Catholic Conference, 1949).

6. Strup et al., The Medical Task Force on Anencephaly. "The Infant with Anencephaly." *NEJM:* 322 (March 8, 1990): 669–74.

7. Kevin O'Rourke and Jean DeBlois, "Induced Delivery of Anencephalic Infants," *Kennedy Institute of Ethics Journal* 4: (March 1994):1.

8. William Daniels, "The Anencephalic Fetus and Termination of Pregnancy," *The Australian Catholic Reporter, XL I (January 1984): 65–74.*

9. Eugene Diamond. "Management of a Pregnancy with an Anencephalic Infant," *Linacre Quarterly* (August 1992): 19–23; Abbot Northwestern Hospital, "Heartbreak Pregnancies" (Minneapolis, Minn., 1993).

10. "Moral Principles Concerning Infants with Anencephaly," *Origins* (October 1996).

About the Center for Health Care Ethics

The Center for Health Care Ethics (CHCE), established in 1979, is a division of Saint Louis University Health Sciences Center (SLUHSC) and serves the people in the schools and hospitals that it comprises. The CHCE helps members of the health care community—primarily at SLU but also throughout the rest of the United States—to recognize and resolve ethical issues in contemporary health care in light of the Catholic ethical tradition. Through teaching, lecturing, and participating in clinical rounds and seminars, the Center's staff provides a consistent framework for understanding and integrating ethical theory and practical application. The CHCE offers an interdisciplinary Ph.D. program in Health Care Ethics in the Catholic tradition, designed to place this tradition in a pluralistic society.

Index

317

reasoned analysis
  collaborative process described, 8–9
  method described, 11–12
Rehnquist, Chief Justice William, 226–27
religious beliefs
  about pain and suffering, 279–80
  on autopsies, 276–78
  and health care, 36–39
  and lifesaving therapy, 113–17
  on playing God, 273–75
  right to refuse treatment, 124–27
  See also Jehovah's Witness
religious faith, 11
renal failure, 13, 53, 99, 100
reproductive technologies
  antifertility drugs, 300–303
  fertility drugs, 307–11
  See also cloning (artificial twinning);
    human embryos, *in vitro*
    fertilization
research. *See* cloning (artificial twinning);
    medical research
Rhodes, L., 36
right to privacy, 234
Roe, Jane, 226, 229
Royce, Josiah, 231

S
Saikewicz case, 49, 51
Saint Louis University Health Sciences
    Center (SLUHSC), 316
schizophrenia, 58
Schweitzer, Arlene, 263, 264
Seed, Richard, 157
Setting Limits (Callahan), 258
Singelenberg, Richard, 114
Smith, Jane, 179
social function/needs, 3, 17
Soelle, Dorothee, 221
somatic cell nuclear transfer (SCNT), 158,
    159, 160
Souter, Justice David, 228
spiritual needs
  as a basic human need, 3
  and creative function, 17
  importance of, 5–6
Spring case, 49, 51
Stevens, Justice John Paul, 227
stewardship concept, 212
Stoics, 205
substitute judgment principle, 55–56
suffering
  defined, 283
  and need for compassion, 282–84
  See also pain

Suffering (Soelle), 221
suicide
  defined, 209
  and myth of "managed death", 208–11
  as a rational choice, 205–8
Supportive Care of the Dying: A Coalition
    of Compassionate Care, 228
surrogate motherhood
  Baby M case, 148, 265
  Schwietzer-Uchytil collaboration,
    263–66

T
Tay-Sachs disease, 147, 151–52
Teel, Judge Charles, 120–21
Teno, Joan, 88
terminal illness, defined, 13
therapeutic research, 58–61, 195, 196
Thomas, Justice Clarence, 222
Thomasma, David, 25
transplantation. *See* bone marrow
    transplant; heart transplant; kidney
    transplant; liver transplant; organ
    donation
truth-telling, in physician-patient
    relationship, 69–71, 285–88
Tuskeegee syphilis study, 61, 195, 306

U
Uchytil, Christa and Kevin, 263
Uniform Definition of Death Act, 180
University of California (Los Angeles)
  Alzheimer's disease study, 61
  schizophrenia study, 58
University of Pittsburgh, Medical Center,
    organ donor protocols, 179, 181

V
vaccine research, 190
value systems
  cultural and religious, 36–39
  and health care reform, 241
  in medical care, 16–19
  patients', 22, 24
  physician-patient conflicts in, 20–21
Veatch, Robert, 139
ventilators, right to remove, 13
vocation, of physicians, 29

W
Wanglie (Helga) case, 127, 128, 129, 132,
    134–37
Washington v. Glucksberg, 234, 235
Webster, William, 121
Winn, Clemintina Geraci, 40–41, 42, 43